SILENT VICTIMS

The Continuing Failure to Protect
Society's Most Vulnerable

The Longcare Scandal

By

John Pring

This HB edition published in the UK and Commonwealth in 2003
by Gibson Square Books Ltd
15 Gibson Square, London N1 0RD
Tel: +44 (0)20 7689 4790; Fax: +44 (0)20 7689 7395
publicity@gibsonsquare.com
www.gibsonsquare.com

UK & Ireland sales by Signature
20 Castlegate, York YO1 9RP
Tel 01904 633 633; Fax 01904 675 445
sales@signaturebooks.co.uk

UK & European distribution by Central Books Ltd
99 Wallis Road, UK London E9 5LN
Tel +44 (0)845 458 9911; Fax +44 (0)845 458 9912
info@centralbooks.com
www.centralbooks.com

Australian
New Zealand,
South Africa,
US sales,
please contact
Gibson Square Books Ltd for contact details.

© 2003 by John Pring

ISBN 1-903933-19-6

The moral right of John Pring to be identified as the author of
this work has been asserted in accordance with the Copyright, Designs
and Patents Act 1988.

All rights reserved. No part of this publication may be reproduced, stored
in a retrieval system, or transmitted, in any form or by any means, electronic,
mechanical, photocopying, recording or otherwise without the prior consent of the
publisher. A catalogue record for this book is available from the Library of Congress
and the British Library.

Printed by Biddles Ltd

Contents

Foreword, by Fiona Mactaggart MP		3
Acknowledgements		9
How It Began		11
Introduction		13

FAMILIES
1	Idiots	19
2	Diagnosis	25
3	Battling the World	29
4	Coping	30
5	Educating Idiots	33
6	School	35
7	Enough is Enough	37
8	Letting Go	38
9	The Perfect Home	42

GORDON ROWE
10	Broadmoor	49
11	Brighton	51
12	From Broadmoor to Somerset	55
13	Like a Zombie	58
14	Sensitive, Able and Caring	63

LONGCARE
15	Welcome to Stoke Place	68

16	Red Apples, Green Apples	70
17	Lottie Perfume	73
18	Gordon's Listening	74
19	Horse Potatoes	79
20	A Walking Christmas Tree	84
21	The Railway Carriages	89
22	Gordon's Girls	92

INVESTIGATIONS

23	Serious Implications	101
24	The Care Staff	105
25	Buckinghamshire County Council	112
26	The Police	124
27	Gordon Rowe	130
28	The Other Visitors	136
29	The Medical Profession	140
30	The Legal System	152
31	The Other Local Authorities	155

AFTER LONGCARE

32	Underwhelmed	169
33	'You Couldn't Hear Anyone Coming'	171
34	'I Want Something Better'	175
35	Ninety Per Cent	180
36	Dorothy	184
37	Rosie	188
38	Greg	191
39	Gary	193
40	Janet	194
41	Nicky	198
42	Simon	206
44	Stefano	210
45	Justice for Longcare Survivors	213
46	An Affront to Human Dignity	216

Epilogue	229
Bibliography	235
Contact details and help-lines	239
Index	240

Foreword

The best writing can create a picture in your mind's eye that engages your interest and makes you want to find out more. I didn't know anything about the issue in this book until I read John Pring's articles. I did not even know there was a home for people with learning disabilities on the outskirts of the town that I came to represent in Parliament. I don't think I am naïve, but I was horrified to learn that, so close to our doorstep, such cruelty was going on. I was shocked that the social workers, inspectors, chiropodists, pharmacists, people who ran voluntary organisations, and others who visited, many of whom served Slough as well as South Bucks and whom I knew, had apparently seen nothing of what was going on. The poorly paid staff who worked at the two Longcare homes did see things that made them worry, but they were intimidated and, without public debate about how to treat people with learning difficulties, many accepted that what they saw was a normal way to behave.

It is harder to write about than many stories because it is about people who are not heard. Not only can many of the characters not speak for themselves, many do not even have contact with any other advocates, friends or family. And it is a story of how horribly easy it is to oppress people who cannot stand up for themselves and who have no-one else to do it for them. It is a story which has changed government policy and the practices of more than one local government body. Readers can learn the lessons which the tale of Longcare has to teach. And it is gruesomely important that we do learn them.

What becomes clear as the pages unfold is not just the casual cruelty and degrading denial of human rights which was the daily experience of people with learning disabilities who lived in Longcare. It is not just the terrible impact on families who discovered that they had entrusted a very vulnerable loved one to the care of a monster who was known to have sexually abused such people before.

But it also becomes clear that we very easily might never have known about it. Even when Buckinghamshire County Council discovered what was happening in a home licensed by them they were concerned to keep the facility going and never showed any interest in making the scandal more widely known so that the lessons could be learnt.

This book is powerful because in it we discover that the people who Gordon Rowe and his accomplices treated so badly are not just silent victims, they have strong personalities, worried families, irritating habits and hopes, fears and anxieties. They cry, they bleed, they get scared. In describing them and in using their own words John Pring provides the antidote to a phenomenon, which he discusses in detail, of society's unwillingness to acknowledge people with learning difficulties, of our reluctance to listen to them and to talk about their needs.

Our silence makes them more vulnerable to abuse, more likely to be victims. While Gordon Rowe, who systematically abused the residents at Longcare, is at an extreme end of the spectrum, there is no doubt that, for someone with learning difficulties, bullying is an everyday experience. This group of people has now become a favoured target of sexual predators frustrated by improved child protection measures.

And just as child abuse used to be a taboo subject this one is still too often taboo. It is rarely discussed and even when abuse is uncovered, justice still fails the victims. Cases are not brought to court, because people with learning disabilities are rarely trusted to be witnesses. Once again we as a society are the ones who silence the victims. And when perpetrators are not prosecuted they often, like Gordon Rowe, go on to abuse again.

I do not think that such abuse could occur, even in the face of someone as dynamic and persuasive as Gordon Rowe, if there were a general social acknowledgement and discussion of the rights of people with learning difficulties. If we lived in a more integrated society where most people have regular experience of sharing our community or workplace with people with learning difficulties things might be different. If the rights of people with learning disabilities were a frequent subject of newspaper articles or public debate, the young employees might have had a moral view, backed by experience, which encouraged them to refuse to deny basic human rights and respect to the residents.

If this book helps in any way to provoke that debate it will probably save lives. The articles that preceded it have already begun to change things for the better. I am grateful to its author for opening my eyes.

Fiona Mactaggart

Member of Parliament for Slough
Under Secretary of State, Home Office

'Wherever there is a human being, I see God-given rights inherent in that being, whatever may be the sex or complexion.'

William Lloyd Garrison (1805-1879)

Author's Note

The accepted terminology used to refer to the type of disability I have written about in Silent Victims has changed many times over the years, including at least six times during the twentieth century alone. This is reflected in Silent Victims, and I apologise for any offence caused by the use of some of these now outdated terms.

The use of an asterisk next to a character's name indicates that it has been changed to protect his or her identity. The residents are referred to by their full name with their permission or that of their guardians. A number of the care staff are referred to by their first name only.

Acknowledgements

This book would not have been possible without the help of hundreds of people over the last nine years. I can't thank them all, but there are some I must mention.

Firstly, my friend Lisa Sherper, who was there throughout. Her wisdom and insights were invaluable, as was her friendship.

Mel Gow's advice, encouragement and friendship were also gratefully received at a time when I needed all three.

I must also thank Martin Rynja, for seeing the importance of the Longcare story, and for sticking with this project for so many years, and Margaret Kennedy, who provided some vital suggestions after reading the draft. I am also extremely grateful to James Clive-Matthews for a fantastic editing job.

Particular thanks are due to Dorothy Thomson, without whom this book would have lost its core. Her courage and selflessness have been a source of constant admiration, as has the unfailing good humour of her husband, Jamie.

But this book would not have happened at all without Janice Raycroft, my first editor, who staked her career on publishing the Longcare story in the Slough Observer back in 1994.

There are many others who have offered help, advice and encouragement over the last nine years, but particular thanks are due to my parents, Rod and Chris Pring, June Raybaud, Nicola Harney and her colleagues at Stewarts, who give lawyers a good name, Fiona Mactaggart MP, who does the same for politicians, everyone at Central England People First, Jenny Bhatia, Neil Morris, Mabel Cooper and everyone at Croydon People First.

Of the many former members of Longcare staff I spoke to, many asked not to be named, but of those who didn't, Clare Johnson deserves particular mention.

Finally, I am incredibly grateful to the families of Gordon Rowe's victims for sharing their stories with me, when it would have been much easier to slam their doors in my face. Particularly Pauline Hennessey, Avril and Brian Scott, Susan and Davyd Power, Benedict Alcindor, Ron and Doreen Deacon, Lidia and Leslie Tunstell and Norma Adams.

And to that one, anonymous, person who sent that leaked document to the *Slough Observer* all those years ago: thank you.

John Pring, London
johnpring@btopenworld.com

How It Began

SIR/MADAM,
FOR OBVIOUS REASONS I AM UNABLE TO SIGN THIS NOTE. HOWEVER, I THINK IT IS AN ISSUE OF SOME IMPORTANCE. THERE APPEAR TO BE SERIOUS IMPLICATIONS, A POSSIBLE COVER-UP, AND NO SIGN THAT OTHER LOCAL GOVERNMENT OFFICES HAVE BEEN NOTIFIED ABOUT THIS MATTER. IT WOULD CERTAINLY WARRANT SOME FURTHER RESEARCH.
SINCERELY,
'CONCERNED'.

It was hand-written in capital letters, dated August 31, 1994, and accompanied by a leaked copy of a Buckinghamshire County Council report written by Jennifer Waldron, head of the council's inspection unit, the department responsible for inspecting residential homes for children, older and disabled people.

The editor of the *Slough Observer*, Janice Raycroft, took one look at the first page of the report, and reached for a cigarette. 'I knew immediately that the bomb had gone off,' she would later say.

A junior reporter with only nine months experience, I was handed the story only because my 'patch' of South Buckinghamshire covered the two homes for adults with learning difficulties referred to in the council document. I had never met anyone with a learning difficulty (the preferred term now for people who used to be called 'mentally handicapped'), other than occasional and fleeting encounters with a few occupants of a residential home in Cheddar, the village where I grew up in Somerset. I had always felt slightly uneasy when passing them on the street; but I never examined my discomfort.

As I began to work on the story, it soon became clear that most of the population shared my ignorance, both of learning difficulties themselves and the multiple levels of victimization that such people endure. I was unprepared, too, for the suffering that would be revealed. But just as unexpected was the resilient integrity and generosity possessed by many of the men and women I came across. They showed me that all human beings, including those we dismiss as unproductive and irrelevant, have the potential to enrich the lives of those around them.

My research eventually began to highlight what it means to have a learning difficulty in Britain today. It became clear that such people have the lowest-paid jobs, if they can find work at all. Their clothes are probably second-hand, their healthcare second-rate and their housing substandard. Most experience a lifetime of petty humiliations and live their lives in unremittingly second-class conditions, their needs and wishes given the lowest priority. Learning disabled people are often hidden away from 'normal' society. If they are lucky enough to live 'in the community', their neighbours resent their presence and ignore them, and they are ridiculed, abused and taken advantage of at every turn.

The story of the report that arrived on my desk at the Slough Observer that day in September 1994 is that of Gordon Rowe, the mental health nurse and later social worker and residential home owner, who over a period of 25 years abused in a depraved and cynical way those for whom he had promised to care. It is also the story of the people who came to live in the three residential homes he was to run, and their families. And it is the story of how these disabled people were let down, discarded, ignored and degraded by society at every turn.

But it is also the story of how others just like them are still being abused today. Many are unable to call for help, and those that do might just as well stay silent.

Today, the social care system seems just as ready to abandon vulnerable adults in residential care. The research in this book suggests that thousands of learning disabled men and women continue to be exposed to possible abuse by living in residential homes far from their families and friends, while receiving none of the regular visits that are supposed to be made by their social workers.

INTRODUCTION

'The extensive investigation which has been carried out has resulted in a considerable body of information which indicates that for many years the homes operated a totally unacceptable regime which meant that a substantial group of vulnerable people were at times denied some of their most basic human rights, as shown in the following paragraphs.

As well as graphic details, the witnesses who made statements almost all expressed feelings of guilt and self-recrimination that they had been powerless to do anything to safeguard and protect residents...

The impression gained is that the prevailing culture was one in which the basic humanity of residents was denied. It is difficult to distil the information given and still convey the enormity and scale of humiliation, deprivation, torment and punishment to which residents were subjected.'

Extract from *Report on Investigation into Allegations of Serious Abuse at Longcare Ltd*—Social Services Department, Buckinghamshire County Council, June 1994

In April 1991, Buckinghamshire County Council recorded the first abuse allegation against Gordon Rowe at Longcare, the residential care company he had set up in the early 80s.

Dorothy Abbott, one of the most able of Longcare's clients, was living in a small flat in the grounds of Stoke Place, one of Rowe's homes, with two other residents, one of whom was her boyfriend, Jimmy. She refused to return from a visit to her sister, claiming Rowe had attacked her.

Dorothy told her social worker how she and her flat-mate, Sylvia, had been about to enjoy an afternoon cup of tea when there was a loud knock at the door. Dorothy knew it was Rowe. She was terrified, because she had been telling staff she was going to 'let it all out what Gordon Rowe was doing to the residents'.

Rowe dragged Dorothy outside 'in caveman style' and threw her to the ground. He stood over her for up to an hour, while she lay bleeding on the cold, wet grass.

Dorothy showed her social worker the healed wound on her hand and made other allegations of poor care—including Rowe pulling residents around and depriving them of meals as a punishment. Dorothy left Stoke Place, but her social worker sent a copy of his report to Buckinghamshire's registration officer, Anthony Barker, and asked whether any other residents, families or social workers had made similar complaints.

Barker agreed the homes were large and regimented, but said he hadn't heard any other such complaints. He visited Longcare to talk to Rowe and his staff. Employees lined up outside Rowe's office, to wait for Barker to interview them. Rowe was pacing up and down next to the queue, warning each of his care workers to 'be careful' what they said. They all knew his office was bugged. The whole episode was a farce.

Even so, during his investigation, Barker received allegations from three former members of staff about over-use of medication at the home, physical assaults and punishments. He also interviewed Dorothy Abbott. She repeated her allegations, and admitted grabbing a pair of scissors to protect herself from Gordon Rowe when he burst into her flat. She also told him four other residents were being ill-treated.

In a letter to Rowe, Barker said: 'I find it difficult to understand why there was so much physical violence when you were dealing with one so physically inferior in both weight and strength.' He drew his attention to various inappropriate methods of 'restraint, discipline or sanctions'. Barker also spoke to Ray Cradock, one of the registered managers of the homes, who told him Longcare was committed to raising standards and that Gordon Rowe was looking to buy a house, so he wouldn't need to live in the grounds.

In the home's regular inspection report the following month, the council said visits would take place every three months, with inspectors monitoring specific areas of care. It also said Longcare should arrange external advice for residents who needed help with their finances, as Dorothy had claimed that Rowe had been taking money from them.

But that was all. There was no full investigation, even though the council was aware Rowe had previously been questioned over allegations of sexual abuse while managing a care home in Somerset eight years earlier.

An investigation finally began on Nov 17, 1993, almost 12 months after the first of a series of anonymous calls by former members of staff to Jennifer Waldron, the head of Buckinghamshire County Council's inspection unit, and more than two and a half years after Dorothy Abbott had been attacked.

The inspection unit interviewed every current and former member of staff they could track down. They interviewed Gordon Rowe and his wife Angela, Ray Cradock and Lorraine Field, another Longcare manager. But they failed to talk to anyone else, including the victims themselves, the residents.

Now, when it seemed as though someone was finally listening, the residents of Longcare had, once again, been denied a voice.

This conclusion was confirmed in May 1995, when the government's Social Services Inspectorate (SSI) uncovered a catalogue of errors and complacency during its inspection of Buckinghamshire's inspection unit (the SSI was performing a routine inspection— it inspects all social services across the country).

The report criticised the unit's failure to talk to residents and relatives during its routine inspection work. It also said it failed to talk to GPs, community nurses and social workers, which, it said, 'served to reinforce the limited contact between residents and the outside community'. The SSI's report concluded that the county council had given a low priority to the inspection unit's work and had granted it insufficient resources when it was set up in 1991.

The council had originally intended to launch the unit with six inspectors and a unit head. Councillors decided instead to cut the number of inspectors to four. According to the Social Services Inspectorate, the county spent less money on social services than any other comparable authority in the country.

It would be reassuring to know that those members of Buckinghamshire's social services committee who had read the inspection unit's disturbing report on Longcare had learned something from that experience. Unfortunately, in February 1996 it emerged that members of that same committee had completed reports on just 29 of the 153 visits they were supposed to have made in 1995 to check on conditions at council-run homes for older people, children and learning disabled clients.

Despite the public exposure of its mistakes, Buckinghamshire County Council—and in particular Jean Jeffrey, its head of social services—refused to admit that they had made any mistakes, or agree to set up an inquiry.

One of those who was convinced a full independent inquiry *was* necessary was Fiona Mactaggart, the newly-elected Labour MP for Slough, whose attention had been drawn to Longcare by the *Slough Observer* shortly before the General Election of 1997. Within days of her election, she wrote to Paul Boateng, the newly-appointed Parliamentary Under Secretary of State at the Department of Health who was responsible for social services, asking him to set up an inquiry. She followed up her letter with a parliamentary question. But Boateng was initially cool on the idea. He thought Bucks could and would learn from its mistakes.

Nonetheless, Boateng agreed to question representatives of Bucks County Council. 'He had a pre-meeting with me and Dominic Grieve [the Conservative MP for Beaconsfield, whose constituency included Stoke Place],' said Mactaggart. 'He said, "this is a lengthy process, we don't necessarily need an inquiry". I had a row with Paul, saying, "you cannot be so feeble. This is serious, we have to find out what's going on." He was intending to rap their knuckles, accept an apology and send them on their way.'

But Jean Jeffrey was not about to be criticised. 'Not only do we have nothing to learn, but our behaviour was exemplary and everyone should learn from us,' she told Boateng.

The minister exploded, said Mactaggart. 'He said, "I'm not being talked to like this," and he just lost it, because of her arrogance. It was her complete refusal to admit that there had been something which was a deep offence to a civilised community for which she was responsible in any way that provoked him into insisting that they have an inquiry, and Paul Boateng angry is quite an interesting sight.'

'I think Paul quite rightly realised as a result of seeing her face to face—which I don't think he had realised before—that there was a serious cultural problem in Bucks social services. He realised that Jean Jeffrey was not going to learn from it unless her nose was rubbed in it. And even when her nose *was* rubbed in it, she didn't.'

The independent inquiry ordered by Boateng was led by Tom Burgner, a retired Treasury official, who in 1996 had written a well-received report into the regulation and inspection of social services. Burgner told me: 'Although we made a lot of recommendations for changes in the law, my over-riding feeling was that if everyone had done their job properly and fully, the duration of the abuse could have been prevented. You can't prevent individual acts of abuse, but this entrenched culture of abuse should never have been allowed. It should have been stopped at source or uncovered sooner. The law gave all the powers. What was lacking was the skill and determination and experience to tackle a difficult case. It was a difficult case for any inspection team to crack, but they made a lot of mistakes.'

'The distinction between what you need to secure a criminal conviction and what you need to challenge a registration—that was not clear in the minds of the inspection unit in 1993 and 1994. Of course, there were also checks that should have been undertaken and information that should have been followed up in 1983, when Stoke Place was first considered for registration.'

Dr Philippa Russell, one of his two colleagues on the Longcare inquiry, said the council should have sought advice from experts, who could have 'asked far more probing questions'. 'Equally, I don't think Buckinghamshire felt competent to actually talk to the residents themselves, or rather question the residents—there's a difference between talking to and questioning.'

'We felt very strongly that during every routine inspection, there should be a proper consultation with the residents, which should be in a private place and should not be with a member of staff sitting in. Now, of course, the residents may or may not tell you that something's going wrong. If they have come from very disadvantaged circumstances they may not know that what is happening is very wrong. But a lot of them will, and at least half of the Longcare residents—if they had been asked—were well able to say what was happening. They knew very, very well. And I think that is actually one of the greatest safeguards—to actually ask people themselves.'

FAMILIES

1. Idiots

> 'The feeble-minded are a parasitic, predatory class, never capable of self-support, or of managing their own affairs... they cause unutterable sorrow at home and are a menace and danger to the community. Feeble-minded women are almost invariably immoral and if at large usually become carriers of venereal disease or give birth to children who are as defective as themselves. Every feeble-minded person, especially the high-grade imbecile, is a potential criminal, needing only the proper environment and opportunity for the development and expression of his criminal tendencies.'
>
> Walter Fernald; speech to Massachusetts Medical Society; 1912

It is only recently that academics have begun to accept that learning disabled people in the Middle Ages were not automatically thrown out onto the streets to fend for themselves, or regarded as offspring of the Devil. Many *were* rejected by their families, usually for reasons of economic survival, but historical documents show legal mechanisms existed to provide for them if their families were unable to do so.

As early as the 14th century a legal distinction was drawn by the Crown between 'idiots' (people with learning difficulties) and 'lunatics' (those with mental health problems). It was an important distinction. Court hearings decided whether a person was one or the other. If an 'idiot', the Crown would act as guardian, taking his property but ensuring his welfare during his lifetime with the proceeds. A lunatic, although treated in a similar way, could reacquire his property if he ever recovered. The courts in the 14th century were therefore aware of the distinctions between mental illness and learning difficulties that many people in the 21st century have still not quite been able to grasp.

Research has also shown that, far from treating idiots as a curse upon their families, they were often seen as having a condition requiring care within and by the community, much as they are today. Parishes were frequently ordered by the courts to arrange for the financial care of those unable to look after themselves.

There were those, like Martin Luther in the 16th century, who believed the birth of an 'idiot child' was a punishment handed down to parents who had committed adultery or did not fear God. Some idiots were put to death. But these cases were rare.

This is not to say that many thousands of disabled people did not end up wandering the highways as thieves and vagabonds or were not forced to turn to prostitution. But throughout the seventeenth and eighteenth centuries, there were mechanisms in place which helped at least some of these people when their family care systems broke down through poverty or death. For instance, the courts administered a system of parochial aid, which they could order to be paid to help idiots receive nursing and lodging with parish nurses. It is unclear how often this safety net was used, but it was there and there is documentary proof that it was used as an early form of community care.

Before the Industrial Revolution, most jobs required only simple skills and were well within the grasp of many 'idiots'. But the process of industrialisation, which began during the eighteenth century, revealed the poor mental dexterity of those with intellectual disabilities. They were relegated to the bottom of the labour market and many became destitute, ending up in workhouses or prisons.

During the 19th century, a new network of workhouses, lunatic asylums, and huge prisons began to spring up. They were organised on a much larger scale than the parish workhouses, private madhouses and local gaols they replaced. Their regimes were harsh and often brutal. They became rejection piles for those who could find no place at the table of a booming, industrialised Britain—elderly paupers, orphans, lunatics and idiots.

Educationalists soon began to wonder whether it might be possible to cure 'mental deficiency', or at least ameliorate its effects in less severely disabled idiots. (Until the end of the nineteenth century, terms such as 'idiot', 'imbecile' and 'feeble-minded' were practically interchangeable. Eventually, they came to classify the severity of the disability: idiots the most profoundly disabled, imbeciles were moderately disabled, and feeble-minded people were those who would now be described as having 'mild' learning difficulties.) Between the late 1840s and the late 1860s, five voluntary institutions for 'educable idiots' were founded in England. They focused on health, nutrition, exercise and 'moral training'. The task was to create 'economically independent and morally competent individuals', and lift the burdens of financial dependency and lifetime care from families.

By 1881, there were about 30,000 classified idiots in institutions in England, but less than 1000 in these specialised idiot asylums. The rest were still in workhouses, lunatic asylums and prisons. Even so, many thousands were still living outside institutions, being cared for in the community, usually by their families.

By the end of the nineteenth century, the mood of optimism about the possibility of educating the 'idiot' had all but evaporated. The country found itself struggling against a perceived tide of vagrancy, crime, prostitution and poverty. The growing numbers of supporters of the eugenics movement used the mentally 'defective' as convenient scapegoats for these social problems. The eugenicist Fernald's speech to the Massachusetts Medical Society in 1912 (quoted at the start of this chapter) is often repeated, but serves to illustrated the attitudes that prevailed among an influential section of opinion-formers.

The idea that such people might be victims of society rather than the cause of its problems did not occur to eugenicists. Instead, they advocated solutions to keep them away from 'decent' people and prevent them reproducing, through confinement, control and rigid segregation of the sexes. Campaigners persuaded Parliament to introduce laws that would certify all those suspected of being 'mentally deficient' and arrange for many of them to be locked away in asylums.

The resulting Mental Deficiency Act of 1913 set the tone for the rest of the century. It gave local authorities two duties: to certify all those considered mentally deficient under the act, and to set up special institutions for those considered not to be receiving adequate care at home. People sent to these institutions, or 'colonies', were expected to work on their farms, or do cleaning, cooking or laundry.

Those in charge of these colonies were often unwilling to discharge members of such a cheap workforce back into the community.

Within a year, the Mental Deficiency Act caused the number of mentally deficient people in these specialised institutions to rise by a third, and between 1916 and 1950, this figure increased from 6,500 to 57,500.

These long-stay 'hospitals' were often brutal places; many were former workhouses. Privacy was non-existent, the regimes harsh and the food poor. Patients often spent their entire day on the ward, if they weren't working in the grounds. Those who did work were not paid, apart from small extra rations. They were locked in, deprived of outside contact. They wore 'uniforms', as if in prison, and the sexes were strictly segregated. Staff training and salaries were poor. Patients were frequently ill-treated. Certification under the Act often meant being confined to a colony for life.

With the launch of the National Health Service in 1948, the long-stay hospitals were transferred into the control of the new hospital authorities, while local authorities kept responsibility for providing services for 'subnormal' people who lived at home.

The Royal Commission of 1954-57 suggested the replacement of institutions with 'community care'. The ideal was a family life environment and the end of segregation. A hostel, or residential or foster home, was the next best thing. The commission said there should be more training centres and sheltered workshops and 'more social support for the mentally handicapped and their families'.

But there was no immediate closing-down of the long-stay hospitals. There were still tens of thousands of people living in these institutions, many of whom had been there for more than fifty years. Instead, under the Mental Health Act of 1959, local authorities were given a duty to provide a range of services and residential accommodation for 'mentally handicapped' people living in the community.

The act also abolished the certification process and replaced the term 'mental deficiency' with the slightly less demeaning 'mental subnormality'. Most patients were now classed as 'voluntary' and were technically free to leave the long-stay hospitals. Some of the more able did so, but were provided with little or no preparation for life in the community. For the hospitals they left, their departure was disastrous: these patients had provided a huge pool of unpaid manual labour, and their loss was an enormous financial blow.

Ten years after the Mental Health Act, the state of long-stay hospitals was summed up by Dr Pauline Morris. Her 1969 survey[1] found 61 per cent of patients living in complexes of more than 1000 beds, only one per cent in single rooms, and 69 per cent in dormitories with space of two feet or less between beds. Only 21 per cent of patients had their own toothbrushes, shaving kit or hairbrushes. Many were living in 'barren conditions', with little occupation and few social relationships. Nearly half of the patients did not receive a single visit in a year.

Dr Morris criticised the 'isolation, cruelty and deprivation of the hospital organisation', but conceded that most members of the public regarded the poor conditions with 'comparative equanimity'. 'Because almost everyone adopts an attitude of untutored pessimism about the possibilities of educating and occupying the handicapped, unjustifiably low standards of care are tolerated,' she wrote.

These low standards were exposed by a string of scandals at long-stay hospitals during the 60s and 70s.

The Ely Hospital Committee of Inquiry reported in March 1969 and concluded that the hospital's regime had been characterised by cruel ill-treatment, inhumane and threatening behaviour towards patients, the pilfering of food and clothes by staff, and indifference by senior staff to complaints. It highlighted overcrowded wards and a lack of privacy for patients, who were allowed few personal possessions. Buildings were old and poorly designed, few patients were discharged, and food and clothing were inadequate. Staff who tried to complain were intimidated into silence. There were poor links with the local community.

The Farleigh Hospital Committee of Inquiry reported two years later. It found that few patients received visits, and even fewer visited anyone outside the hospital. In one ward, nearly all of the residents never left the room. There was a lack of space, equipment and staff, and a 'harmful over-use of drugs'. Suspicious deaths were not reported to the coroner. Three nurses were eventually jailed for ill-treating patients.

These scandals forced the Government to set up the Hospital Advisory Service (HAS), to inspect and improve the long-stay hospitals. The HAS was abolished in 1975, when acceptable minimum standards were supposedly reached. But the scandals continued as before.

In May, 1974, the Report of the Committee of Inquiry into South Ockendon Hospital again found worryingly poor standards of nursing care. The inspector blamed poor management and problems with the handling of complaints. The hospital, he said, was overcrowded and understaffed. Among other things, he blamed a lack of funding. Staff tended to rely on tranquillisers, rather than providing activities, to control the patients. Side-rooms on wards were used as punishment areas for patients who didn't 'behave' or co-operate with staff. Often, there would be just a mattress and blanket on the floor of these punishment rooms.

The Committee of Inquiry into Normansfield Hospital in November, 1978, was not about cruelty to patients, but still found that 'the standard of nursing care was generally extremely low'. There was too much use of seclusion of 'difficult' patients. Hospital buildings were neglected and dangerous and patients were sometimes soaked as they slept, because of leaky roofs. Faeces and urine were frequently left unattended for days. The inspector concluded that the hospital was 'generally speaking, filthy', the wards bare and reminiscent of workhouses. Patients had no personal possessions and no privacy.

In 1971, the Conservative government had produced its White Paper, *Better Services for the Mentally Handicapped*. Its aim had been to address the poor state of services for people with learning difficulties and explain why the government felt there needed to be a greater emphasis on care in the community and less on care in hospital. The Department of Health and Social Security also hoped that its white paper might lead to greater public understanding of learning disabled people.

When it was published in June 1971, the white paper had drawn detailed attention to overcrowding, unsuitable buildings, poor living standards and chronic under-staffing in existing residential services. The government said it would make extra resources available, and expected hospital boards to reallocate money to long-stay hospitals. Either this money hadn't been enough, or the boards hadn't been entirely committed to the idea of spending scarce resources on 'mentally handicapped' people. Many patients were still living in squalor.

But it wasn't just about money. Reginald Johnson, of the Richmond Society for Mentally Handicapped Children, told the Normansfield inquiry eight years after the White Paper: 'A number of patients at Normansfield are patients there because their families simply could not cope... It is difficult for us to see that there is adequate co-operation between education, social services and health authorities... If there were more support services for parents of children at home, then I think it probable that a great many more parents would be able to keep their children at home.'

The White Paper had emphasised the importance of different agencies working together. But the subsequent failure to do so by health authorities and social services, and this lack of support for parents, would combine to produce conditions where appalling levels of abuse could thrive.

[1] *Put Away: A Sociological Study of Institutions for the Mentally Retarded*, by Dr Pauline Morris.

2. Diagnosis

> 'One man from Wales said: "I live on a council estate. Kids, a group of four or five children, abuse me all the time. One of them has threatened to beat me up when I leave the home to visit my sister. I fancy moving as I can't go on. I cry about it. They make fun of me, they throw stones, they smash my windows. Last year, our gate was broken, and somebody smashed all the glass windows in our greenhouse. The police won't do anything about it."'
>
> Mencap; *Living in Fear*, June 1999

Many doctors and nurses believed—and many still do—that children born with a 'mental handicap' were nothing but a burden on society, their families and the NHS. There were in practise two choices for parents: have your child put away in a long-stay hospital, or take him or her home and do your best—on your own—to look after him or her. But don't expect much advice or support from the medical profession.

Janet

The family GP told Irene Ward she was just being over-anxious. There's nothing to worry about, he said, your daughter is perfectly OK. But she knew something was wrong. There was something in the way her daughter moved, the noises she made. She had four perfectly healthy children already; she could see the difference. She kept taking Janet back to the doctor, but he told her to be patient. 'She'll be fine,' he said. 'She's just a little slow.' He refused to refer Janet to a specialist. It was 1968.

As the weeks and months passed, Irene became ever more convinced that something was wrong. Eventually, after repeated requests, she was referred to Great Ormond Street Hospital for Children in London. After Janet was examined, Irene was given a letter to hand to her GP.

Irene's daughter Pauline remembers sitting in her aunt's kitchen, watching her mother and her aunt discuss what to do with the letter. They finally decided to steam it open.

'The letter said Janet would not be able to walk or talk, that she would be a vegetable,' says Pauline. 'My mum was crying, she was absolutely hysterical. It was just a terrible way to find out.'

Tests had revealed that Janet was 'mentally retarded and epileptic'. While she was in the womb, the umbilical cord had become wrapped around her neck, interrupting the blood supply to her brain, leaving it permanently damaged.

Greg

By the time she gave birth to Greg, her sixth child, in February 1965, Norma Adams also knew something about bringing up babies. So when she noticed that her son didn't seem to be interested in toys and wasn't 'babbling' the way her other children had, she knew something was wrong. Physically, Greg was fine—he was crawling around faster than any of the others at his age—but Norma's intuition told her he was different.

When she took Greg to her GP, he laughed at her. 'With your experience, you should know all babies progress at different speeds,' he said.

'No,' she said, 'with my experience that's exactly why I know something is wrong.' Despite her protests, he refused to refer Greg to a specialist.

When Greg was 11 months old, the family moved to a different part of London. Norma immediately visited the family's new GP. She examined Greg and told Norma she could see nothing wrong, but arranged for him to see a specialist.

Norma's suspicions were soon confirmed. Greg was hyperkinetic—a condition which meant that he rarely stopped moving—and 'mentally handicapped'.

Nicky

Nicky Power had been born a normal, healthy baby on January 17, 1967.

Eleven months later, on Boxing Day, her parents Susan and Davyd took her to spend the day with Susan's mother and step-father in Maidstone. When they woke Nicky up that evening, she appeared to be developing a cold. By the time they had driven back to their home in nearby Tonbridge, Nicky was unconscious and her right side paralysed. She was rushed to hospital and the Powers were told she might not make it through the night. At one stage, her temperature reached 109 degrees. But she survived.

'Thirty years ago, meningitis wasn't really heard of,' says Susan. 'We didn't know the symptoms or realise how rapidly it came on. It all happened within about two hours.' Davyd and Susan believed Nicky had made a full recovery.

But they soon became worried. Nicky would do nothing but sit screaming and rocking on the floor for hours at a time.

Susan and Davyd took her back to the hospital when she was 18 months old. Nicky was quite calm at first, but as the doctor started to examine her, she began screaming and bashing her head against the wall. The doctor said: 'Is this what you mean?' He told them to leave the room. A few minutes later, he called them back in and said: 'The best thing you could do is put her in a home, because she will only ever be a year old.'

The Powers had been handed a piece of information that would change their lives. Unfortunately, the ignorance demonstrated by this doctor was only a taster of what was to come. 'I came home just in a heap,' says Susan. 'My worst fears had been confirmed.'

It was only when they paid to see a consultant in London a fortnight later that they were told what was wrong. After examining their daughter, he asked them: 'You realise that your daughter is severely brain damaged?' He said he would write to Kent County Council to arrange for Nicky to attend a special school.

Stefano

Stefano Tunstell was born on October 31, 1967. At first, he seemed like any other baby. He talked and smiled and seemed to like people. But, from the age of about thirty months, he started to become withdrawn. His parents Lidia and Leslie became more and more concerned as Stefano slowly began to lose the speech he had learned.

Lidia was making frequent trips to see her parents in Italy and it was an Italian doctor who advised her to take Stefano to a psychologist. However, when she returned to England, the family GP assured her there was nothing wrong with her son. It was only when she returned to Italy when Stefano was four that she was able to take him to a specialist. By this time she was becoming 'a little desperate'. She knew something was wrong. The psychologist told her Stefano had 'an autistic tendency', but that it was not yet that serious.

'He felt that with the right sort of help, Stefano would be able to come back to normality,' says Lidia. 'He had been such a sociable little baby—

we never thought he was going to become so disabled.'

The causes of autism are still unclear, although genetic and biological factors are both believed to play a part. No two autistic people are the same, but all share difficulties in using language, understanding social relationships, and using their imagination, and have a tendency to repeat familiar routines.

On their return to England, Stefano was taken to a GP. 'She saw Stefano and she was absolutely horrible,' says Lidia. 'She kept saying, 'It's very odd. It's very odd. He ought to go to a special school.' I felt completely devastated, because he wasn't odd, he was backward.'

Gary

Ron Deacon, too, was to discover that once you became a parent of a 'mentally handicapped' child, the National Health Service was a much less welcoming place.

He was 56 when his step-daughter, Angela, asked him for help. It was April, 1968, and she had just given birth to a son, Gary. Angela told Ron there was no way she could look after her baby—she had no idea who the father was, and her fiancé was refusing to marry her if Gary was part of the package.

Ron and his wife agreed to look after Gary at their home near Maidenhead. He appeared at first to be a healthy baby, although he had problems sleeping and cried a lot. When Angela asked Ron to adopt her son, when he was just a few months old, he agreed.

Ron said later: 'Angela's fella made it quite plain that he would not accept Gary, and I thought he would end up being adopted or going to a home. I didn't want that to happen.

But I wasn't that young and I was worried the courts wouldn't accept me.' But they did, and Ron became Gary's legal father.

As Gary grew older, the Deacons realised he wasn't learning how to chew solid foods. Ron would take him down to his local pub, and sit in the garden, encouraging him to copy his actions as he chewed on a mouthful of crisps. Gary was also still not sleeping well, and Ron would often put him in the back of his car in the early hours of the morning and drive up the M4 motorway to Heathrow Airport to lull him to sleep.

As the months passed, Ron and his wife became increasingly concerned at Gary's slow development. They took him to their local GP, who finally told them the truth: Gary was autistic and 'mentally handicapped', due to brain damage at birth. The medical authorities had known about Gary's condition, but had decided not to tell them. Ron had struggled to bring up his young son for nearly two years without the benefit of any specialist advice.

All five families were learning quickly how wide was the gulf between the love that parents feel for their 'mentally handicapped' son or daughter and the way the outside world views that child.

3. Battling the World

> 'The Royal Commission [1957]... recommended that... hospitals should be responsible only for those requiring specialist medical treatment or training or continual nursing supervision.'
>
> 'The aim should be to fix for each area as early a date as possible after which the hospitals will not be asked to admit any more people who need residential rather than hospital care.'
>
> Government White Paper,
> *Better Services for the Mentally Handicapped*, June 1971
>
> 'The Government will enable all people currently living in long-stay hospitals to move into more appropriate accommodation by April 2004.'
>
> Government White Paper, *Valuing People:
> A New Strategy for Learning Disability for the 21st Century*,
> March 2001

After 1971, the year the government announced in its White Paper that the huge, long-stay hospitals should gradually be closed down and replaced by residential homes, the hospitals remained overcrowded. The demand for places in residential homes was already seven times higher than supply, so most parents of 'mentally handicapped' children kept them at home, but were offered little or no support to do so. The White Paper had admitted that many families were 'under almost unbearable stress' and received little 'practical help and advice' to deal with it. Little would be done over the next 30 years to address this problem.

Most of the right words had been there in the White Paper, just as they had been there in the report of the Royal Commission in 1957. What had been missing was the political will to fund those words. In addition, Social Services departments placed 'mentally handicapped' people way down their list of priorities. As one social worker put it later: 'Much of social work was taken up with the logistics of childcare, so the mentally handicapped person—who wasn't deemed able to grow and develop as a person—was not a high priority.'

Faced with such obstacles, the parents of a 'mentally handicapped' child felt they were battling against the world. But few realised what was the danger they would be exposing their child to by placing her in a residential home.

4. Coping

> 'I've been raped five times by different people. People think that we're an easy target, that's why they abuse people with learning disabilities, and I think that's all wrong.'
>
> 'Kate'; speaking on File On 4; Radio Four; June 11, 2002

Irene Ward was determined not to give up on Janet, despite the gloomy conclusions reached by the 'experts'. She could not bear the thought of her daughter being sent away to a home. Her family was concerned at the extra burden, but Irene was ready to fight, and so was Janet. By the age of four, Janet had learned to walk. By the age of five, she could say the words 'mum' and 'dad'.

Janet's father, Tony, had married Irene when he was young, and relied heavily on her. When Janet was diagnosed as having a 'mental handicap', the family worried about how he would cope, but Janet changed him almost overnight. Unlike his other children, Janet was never punished with a smack, and he never raised his voice when she misbehaved. He celebrated the slightest progress in her development.

Janet's older brother and sisters spent many hours playing with her, helping her to learn skills of speech and dexterity the specialists had never believed possible. But they paid a price for having Janet around.

Pauline, who was six years older than Janet, says: 'Janet was happy and active, but she was very, very demanding of my mother. My other sister was only two years older than Janet, but none of us could sit on mum's lap or hold her hand. She would just drag us off.'

The family could never relax. Janet only had to see an open door and she was through it. After an incident on holiday in which Janet had fallen from a first-floor balcony while Pauline was looking after her, Irene put locks on all the windows and doors at home.

Despite such restrictions, Pauline never resented Janet. She and her siblings were very protective of her. 'She used to have one of those disabled buggies with blue and white stripes. Everybody used to stare wherever we went—adults and children. One day, I was pushing her in the pushchair with my sister, and some children from my school saw us and started laughing and shouting 'spastic'. I let go of Janet to try and chase after them, but she leaned forward and fell out. She had a lump the size of an egg on her face. I got a real telling off from mum.

'We weren't ashamed of her, we were embarrassed. When you start courting and you bring your boyfriends home and your sister is always between you… Most long-term friends got on well with her, but we probably kept new boyfriends out of the way for a while.'

The Powers would also discover that having a 'mentally handicapped' child would change their lives.

'We found out who our friends were,' says Susan. 'They would ask: 'How's Nicola?' and I would say: 'Just the same' and they would say: 'I can't stand it when she screams.' We lost contact with a lot of people, including her god-mother.'

There were no special nurseries or playgroups, Susan didn't know anybody in a similar situation and she knew nothing about her daughter's impairment. The authorities were not interested. All the Powers were given was a prescription for a strong sedative that left Nicky so drugged up she would do nothing all day but sit on the floor, rocking backwards and forwards.

Norma Adams had problems of a different kind. Even now, more than 30 years later, she remembers vividly what it was like trying to cope with a child who wouldn't sit still for a minute.

'By the time he had turned two, he was so active, he never stopped, never sat down, never stopped moving from the moment his eyes were open. And he didn't walk, he ran. He didn't sleep, except for short half-hour naps totalling maybe four or five hours in every 24, which meant I didn't sleep. I had other children at home, so it was a pretty stressful time.'

Even though Norma was only grabbing a couple of hours of uninterrupted sleep a day, the authorities were unwilling to help. Greg was her responsibility, they told her.

Simon

Simon Scott had been born disabled, but his parents believed it was an impairment they could manage. Avril and Brian Scott tried to treat him as an equal to his brothers and sisters, and bring him up with children his own age, but he was just too different.

Simon was a 'happy little soul' and would sit and play with his toy cars all day, stopping for nothing except food. 'Otherwise, he didn't do a lot,' says his dad, 'he was very slow walking and talking and one of his hands hung down. He had his tantrums, and when nothing went right, he got frustrated and everything went, but he was good and he was happy.' Yet Simon still needed nearly 24 hours a day care and an uninterrupted night's sleep for his parents was unheard of.

He later attended a special school close to home. 'He couldn't cope with a lot of children running around, because he couldn't keep up with them,' says Avril. 'He got frustrated.' Simon seemed to take in the lessons he was taught, but found it difficult to apply this knowledge. 'He would sit and listen to you and absorb what you were saying, but it was expressing his feelings he couldn't do,' she says.

When he was about six, Simon started having epileptic seizures. Many learning disabled people are susceptible to epilepsy, a condition in which the brain is struck by sparks of internal electricity, causing seizures or convulsions, during which they can lose consciousness. Simon's seizures became so lengthy and frequent that, when he was 16, he spent more than a year at an epilepsy hospital. His parents eventually withdrew him after a doctor failed to diagnose a serious infection in his ankle, and he nearly had to have the leg amputated.

Simon returned home, and spent two years at another epilepsy hospital in Buckinghamshire to try to stabilise his condition.

Despite his medical problems, Simon was always ready with a cheeky grin. Just over five feet tall, he was full of energy and a handful for whoever was caring for him. He was, Brian says now, a typical 'bolshie' teenager.

Ron Deacon was soon learned that no-one would be there to help him look after Gary. His wife did not cope well with Gary's impairment, and after she died when he was five, the pressure on Ron intensified.

Even when Gary began attending a special school a few miles from their home near Maidenhead, there was no time for Ron to relax. His day began by waking, washing and dressing his son, and making breakfast. Then he would see him into a taxi, before heading off to work as a taxi driver himself. Later, a friend would meet Gary from another taxi after school, and Ron would return home to make dinner and do the other chores, before preparing Gary for bed. A kind neighbour helped with some of the housework, but it wasn't enough. Ron couldn't relieve the stress by talking to his son in the evenings, because Gary would only ever learn to say 'yes' or 'no'. Instead, father and son would watch television, and Ron began to drink heavily. Eventually, he had a nervous breakdown.

'People who have normal children don't realise what it's like,' he says. 'There are times when you feel as though your head is going to explode with frustration, because you just don't know what to do next.'

5. Educating Idiots

'More than two thirds of people would be unhappy to see a child with a learning disability or mental health problem alongside non-disabled pupils in a classroom, according to a new survey.'

Disability Now, January 2002

Following the introduction of universal compulsory education in the 1870s, it soon became clear that teachers were ignoring feeble-minded and physically disabled children and concentrating instead on brighter pupils. But it was not until 1892 that the first special schools opened, following a report by the Royal Commission on the Blind and Deaf which concluded that mentally deficient children should not remain in workhouses or lunatic asylums and that local authorities should educate them.

By 1896, there were 24 special schools in London, attended by over 900 children, and others run by school boards in Nottingham, Birmingham, Bristol, Bradford and Brighton. But the eugenics movement was slowly becoming more influential. Its followers demanded segregation and sterilisation. The use of intelligence testing was a key weapon, used to argue that children who achieved poor results would never be able to improve, and that expenditure on education could only be justified as preparatory training for more permanent, institutional care.

Following pressure from supporters of the eugenics movement, both from the Fabian Society and Conservatives, the government established the Royal Commission on the Care and Control of the Feeble-Minded in 1904 to assess the issue. It sat for four years and heard evidence on the role of special schools and the relationship between mental defects and crime, drunkenness, poverty, prostitution and illegitimacy. When it finally reported, it recommended that early schooling should develop into industrial training and that an institutional system was superior to the special school system.

The Mental Deficiency Act 1913 gave Education Authorities the duty of deciding which children aged between seven and sixteen were deficient and incapable of being educated in special schools. These children were to be passed on to the mental deficiency committees and were given brief and superficial intelligence tests to justify the decision to send them to an institution. No account was taken of the possible effects of prolonged hospital care, a family bereavement, poverty or physical disability on a child's development.

This certification process—often condemning children to a lifetime of care in long-stay hospitals—was not abolished until the Education Act of 1944, which obliged local education authorities to provide special education. The 1944 act also set out 11 categories of disabled children, with the aim of avoiding the rigid separation of disabled and non-disabled, and replaced the use of the term 'mentally deficient' with 'educationally subnormal'. Civil servants suggested the term should apply to children 20 per cent or more below average ability.

In 1970, the Education (Handicapped Children) Act 1970 forced local education authorities to provide education for all 'mentally handicapped' children. Until then, the more severely disabled children had been excluded from the education system set up under the 1944 Act—those who lived at home had been the responsibility of local authorities' health departments, while hospital authorities had looked after children who lived in long-stay hospitals.

Although there were wide variations between different authorities, and hundreds of children were on waiting lists for special schools, these were at least small steps towards providing some kind of education for learning disabled children.

6. School

> 'Hilary Cooke, who has a learning disability, was about to step on to a bus when the driver said: 'I don't want you on this bus—you make me feel sick.' Recalling the incident, she says: 'He shut the door right in my face and drove off. I felt numb. Other times, children in the street have called me names, like "spastic" or "fatty". I do try not to take notice, but it's hard, very hard.'
>
> *The Guardian*, 'Society' section, April 3, 2002

The local authority's attitude to Greg Adams changed abruptly the day the social services department learned he was autistic, at the age of four. The condition had first been recognised by the medical profession only about 20 years before and research was still in its infancy. However, the London Borough of Hammersmith and Fulham's social services department had its own day nursery with a specialist unit for autistic children and was happy to accept Greg.

In the few hours he spent at the nursery, his mother had to try and pack in everything else in her life: shopping, cooking, cleaning. She also had five teenage children still living at home, including two step-children. They needed their mother, too.

Greg stayed at the nursery until he was five. He was still only sleeping an hour at a time and would then be awake for the next two hours. He was a loner, but—compared to some autistic children—didn't mind being with other people; he simply ignored them. As long as he had plenty of space to run in, he was happy. Greg didn't cry, or throw tantrums. He just wanted to be on the move.

But the stress and sleepless nights were taking their toll on his mother. 'I had had enough. I just couldn't take any more,' says Norma. 'I really felt I couldn't take any more. I asked if he could be taken into care for two or three weeks, so I could have a break. I had quite a battle, but eventually I got social services to agree. After that, he went away for a short period every year and I went away on holiday.'

*

Stefano Tunstell's schooling began promisingly. The head of the local primary school in Epsom, Surrey, said Stefano could attend her mainstream school. But when she left a few weeks later, the new head told the Tunstells there wouldn't be room for him anymore. After just six weeks, Stefano had to leave his new school.

He moved to a special school and progressed well at first, but soon began to react badly to the strict regime. 'He was always upset and he would come home crying. Often, he would be sick and vomiting,' his mother, Lidia, remembers.

She decided to take Stefano back to Italy to see the psychologist who had first diagnosed his autism. He told her the Epsom school was 'absolutely the wrong environment' for her nine-year-old son, but that it was not too late to help him.

Lidia decided to remove Stefano from the school. After a visit to a Harley Street specialist, and a long fight with the local education authority, Lidia and her husband Leslie, a local government officer, were allowed to move Stefano to an assessment unit at Queen Mary's Hospital for Children, in Carshalton. He seemed happier there and began to make progress.

But the unit only took children until they were 12, and Stefano soon had to move again. 'It was a nightmare looking for somewhere for him, because Surrey County Council weren't doing anything,' says Lidia. 'There was no support from social workers. They were very unkind and insensitive. There wasn't any awareness of the situation and the hurt that having a child like Stefano was causing. It was almost as if Stefano had died and we had to cope with a different child.'

They also had to deal with other people's attitudes to their son. 'People were not very sympathetic. He looks so normal and then all of a sudden he might do something like shout or pick up something he shouldn't do and get into a temper if he can't have it. You never know what he is going to do next. Other people would say: "These parents do not have any control over their children."'

Stefano moved to a boarding school for autistic children in Hampshire, and stayed there for four years. When he had to leave at sixteen, his parents battled with Surrey to pay for him to attend St Margaret's School in Croydon, run by The Spastics Society (now renamed Scope).

He had 'one of the best years of his life' at St Margaret's, but when it closed down, Stefano had to move again.

By now the Tunstells were used to fighting for their son, persuading the education authority to pay for him to attend schools that could cater for his needs. But it was always left to them to find him the most appropriate school. Lidia, a college languages tutor, told me: 'It was a nightmare, because every time we suggested somewhere, it was always too expensive, and there was nowhere suitable for him to go in Surrey. It took ages every time he had to move.'

She was not to know that the family's nightmare was only just beginning.

7. Enough is Enough

> 'Millions of pounds intended for services for people with learning disabilities has been spent on other things by cash-strapped strategic health authorities... there will be embarrassment at the failure to follow through the spirit of *Valuing People*, the learning disability white paper published in 2001. Discomfort in Westminster and Whitehall will be all the more acute because the government will fail to meet its target of closing the remaining English long-stay hospitals for learning disabled people by next spring.'
>
> *The Guardian*, 'Society' section, July 30, 2003

During the 70s, the number of private residential homes rapidly expanded. Many were set up by well-meaning people looking to create caring environments. But there was serious money to be made, and many others—businessmen, social workers, nurses, anyone with a few thousand pounds to invest in a property—were simply scrabbling to get their hands on a slice of the pie.

The movement towards community care had accelerated in the 60s, following the Royal Commission and the growing realisation that living in an institutional environment was harmful. But for many former patients, it was merely a move from a large institution to a smaller one. Many of the residential homes they moved into were more like long-stay hospitals than the family-type homes campaigners were advocating.

Yet the sector was also expanding far too slowly to cope with demand. At the start of the 70s, many parts of the country had few facilities for residential care outside the long-stay hospitals, plus a shortage of social and care workers. The 1971 White Paper found there were about 4,300 places in residential homes, compared with a need for nearly 30,000.

8. Letting Go

> 'Other authorities were pessimistic about their ability to influence the quality of care. One education officer reported: "A little while ago we did look at imposing a contract on placements which would make them write down all sorts of stuff about the qualifications of their staff and their staff ratios and all the rest of it. I don't think we've pursued that. Part of the problem is that it's a seller's market. If you are there with a difficult to place youngster you don't start saying 'oh by the way will you now fill in this form in triplicate.'"
>
> David Abbott, Jenny Morris and Linda Ward,
> *Disabled Children and Residential Schools:*
> *A Study of Local Authority Policy and Practice*,
> Norah Fry Research Centre, 2000

Over the previous century, the motives for placing a 'mentally handicapped' relative in residential or institutional care have hardly changed. David Wright, in an article on attitudes to idiots and imbeciles in Victorian England,[1] found that parents trying to have children admitted to an asylum talked about the problems their children had with feeding, dressing, toileting and self-care. They described how their sons and daughters wandered out alone at night, talked to strangers, or even 'leapt at the legs of a passing horse'.

The frustrations and difficulties of caring for a 'mentally handicapped' child have probably not really changed from even earlier times. And without the necessary help and support from the authorities, there will nearly always come a time when parents—no matter how much they love their child—will say: 'Enough is enough. I can't take any more.'

When Janet was five, she began to attend a special school. Her mother joined her one day a week. Janet was extremely hyperactive, never slept more than four or five hours a night, and could never be left alone when awake. But Irene refused even to seek respite care, to allow herself a break: Janet was her daughter and she was determined that she was going to take care of her.

But by the age of eight, Janet had become even more difficult to care for. Her epileptic seizures had become more frequent, and she needed more care and stimulation than the family could provide. Although the thought of putting her daughter in a home still terrified Irene, she realised residential care was the only sensible option, and Janet began a new life at a residential convent school in Hertfordshire for children with epilepsy and 'mental handicaps'.

'Mum felt very, very guilty. She felt that she should have been able to cope, but she knew the opportunities for Janet were much greater than she could have provided,' says Pauline.

Although it was tough for the family to let her go, they immediately noticed the difference at home. 'It wasn't until she went into residential care that we realised what real family life should be like,' says Pauline. 'It was like a whole new experience. It was the peacefulness of it most of all. Janet was very demanding and wanted to be amused all the time. After a couple of weeks, we felt immensely relieved that we had reality. It was much more relaxed. Mum seemed a lot healthier. She wasn't so tired. We did miss Janet, but there was also a relief every time she went back after a visit home.'

Despite her mother's fears, Janet was happy in her new home, surrounded by children her own age. She learned new skills like horse-riding, dancing and swimming, and attended full-time lessons. She made a lot of friends and often seemed annoyed when she had to return home. She learned to read simple words and perform basic sums. Her confidence grew. Soon, even Irene began to realise the move had been the right one.

There were frequent trips home: at weekends, holidays, birthdays. Janet was a bridesmaid at Pauline's wedding. And when Pauline had children of her own, Janet enjoyed teaching them to say 'please' and 'thank you' when they came to visit. Then Janet turned eighteen, and her life changed again.

As an adult, Janet had to leave the classes and her childhood behind and join the adult section of the home. There were no more riding lessons. Instead, she was given chores around the house. Most of her days were spent sitting in a chair, surrounded by far more severely disabled people. Janet kept trying to visit her friends at the other end of the building. She was desperately unhappy.

*

With the Powers, the decision to resort to residential care took slightly longer, but was just as inevitable.

As the years passed, it had become harder and harder for them to cope with Nicky, especially for Susan, who took the full brunt of her 13-year-old daughter's tantrums. They became so bad that Nicky was beating her mother up, punching her and pulling her hair, frustrated at her inability to communicate and understand social skills like learning to dress herself and comb her hair. Susan was on the verge of a nervous breakdown. She and Davyd talked to their social worker, who told them they had to think of their son, who was studying for his A-levels. She advised them to send Nicky to a boarding school. Susan wanted to 'plod on' with things the way they were, but the social worker told her: 'You have had her for 12 years. You deserve a break. You can't continue the way things are.' Susan and Davyd decided she was right and asked for help from Kent County Council. They had to appear before a tribunal, to explain why they wanted to send their daughter away. The council eventually agreed that Nicky could spend twelve months at a boarding-school, until their son finished his A-levels.

After Nicky had been at the school about six months, Susan received a telephone call from one of her teachers. She told Susan they were having terrible problems coping with Nicky, and she would probably never be able to return home to live with her parents. The school agreed she could stay with them until she was old enough to move to an adult home.

'It caused me terrible heart-break,' says Susan. 'The whole thing is like living through a nightmare and it doesn't get any better, because you can't see an end to it.'

Lidia and Leslie Tunstell also knew they would soon have to hand Stefano over into someone else's full-time care.

Stefano had spent eighteen months at a school in Telford, when his social worker finally gave his parents the news they had been dreading: their son was twenty years old and it was too expensive to keep him at a specialist school. Surrey's education authority was passing responsibility for him to social services. Stefano would have to be found a place at a care home.

Although they were concerned, Lidia and her husband believed residential care would be in Stefano's best interests. 'We put our extremely vulnerable child in a home, not because we wanted to get rid of him, but because we thought maybe they could help him and he would mix with other people,' she says. 'I was very worried, extremely uneasy, but he had reached the level where he couldn't go to school. We felt he needed more space and I felt selfish for wanting to keep him at home.'

Ron Deacon was now in his early 70s, a single parent, recovering from a nervous breakdown and caring for Gary on his own. Eventually, his social worker suggested that Ron should consider residential care for his son.

Gary had reached sixteen, a bright-eyed, dark-haired teenager. He had reached the age at which he would have to leave Holyport Manor, and no other school could find a place for him. Ron decided to accept his social worker's advice.

'I was very upset about it, but I was getting on in years and I knew that, if something happened to me, being a one-parent family, Gary could have been stuck anywhere,' says Ron. 'I was relieved for myself, but it was very emotional. It's not nice having to part with your son.'

Norma Adams, too, was approaching the moment when she would have to make the decision to send her child away. But nothing could have prepared her for how difficult that decision would be.

When Greg was five, he was transferred to a special care unit, which meant he was away from home for slightly longer periods every day. He stayed there for two years, until a new school for autistic children opened in Hammersmith.

Greg spent the next four years there, but the family lived at the opposite end of the borough and the head teacher became increasingly concerned that so much of Greg's life was being wasted on the traffic-clogged streets of west London. She told Norma she should consider a boarding school.

It was a terrible decision to have to make. 'I was very definitely split over it,' says Norma. 'The practical side of me said 'yes, yes, yes', and the mothering side of me said 'no, no, no', but I knew it was the right thing to do. I knew I was too emotionally involved in him to teach him all he should be taught and could be taught. Even to this day, in a funny sort of way, there are two of me where Greg is concerned. A tiny bit of my heart will not accept there is something wrong with him. Who wants to accept there is something wrong with their lovely baby boy? But I always let my practical side rule in the end.'

A Mencap friend told her about a new unit for autistic children opening at Great Stony School in Ongar. Despite officers from Greater London Council trying to persuade her that the unit was both non-existent and already full, she eventually convinced them to accept Greg.

Greg was at Great Stony until he was fourteen and seemed to be doing well. But then GLC decided to change the format of the school and, instead of admitting only 'mentally handicapped' children, decided to mix in a few 'delinquents'. Norma decided there was no way she was going to let her son mix with young tearaways, and arranged for him to be moved to Bradstow School, in Broadstairs, Kent. He was there for two years until, at the age of 16, Norma was told it was time for him to begin life as an adult.

Norma had been a physical training instructor. She enjoyed walking and running, but, at nearly sixty years old, was finding it harder to keep up with her son. By now he was a strapping teenager.

'He was a climber, an escaper. I thought that if I had him home, which was what my heart was telling me to do, I would give myself another five years, top whack, and then I would be dead. Then who would look after him? If I let him go into permanent residential care, I was going to live a lot longer and would be able to keep tabs on him, make sure everything went all right. It was very difficult, though. I felt as though I was rejecting him.'

[1] Wright, David: *Childlike in his Innocence: Lay Attitudes to 'Idiots' and 'Imbeciles' in Victorian England.*

9. The Perfect Home

'All the research shows that people, generally speaking, abuse people they judge more vulnerable than themselves. And the message they are getting at the moment from our legal system right the way through is, basically, if they abuse people with a learning disability, the chances are they'll get away with it.'

David Congdon, Mencap, *File on 4*, Radio 4; June 11, 2002

It was Greg's class teacher at Bradstow who told Norma about Gordon Rowe and The Old Rectory, a new residential home that was not yet full. She sent off for a brochure and was impressed with its rural setting and wide range of activities, therapists and trained staff. It talked about providing a 'constructive way of life for mentally handicapped adults' and helping residents develop their potential. 'Our staff,' Rowe wrote, 'will be expected to be aware that the resident needs to feel cared about as well as cared for.'

Norma visited the home—in a small village in Somerset's Quantock Hills—with Greg's social worker, and met both Gordon Rowe and his assistant Angela Adams. Norma liked Gordon but had reservations about Angela. She says it was just an instinct. They asked Gordon about the promised activities and therapists—of which there were no signs—and were told the services would all be up and running when the home was full.

'It was a heart-rending decision,' says Norma. 'It was quite a long way to The Old Rectory and I felt as though I was rejecting Greg. I still do to a degree. There is always the mother side of me that wants him with me and wants to look after him, and the practical side that wants to do what is best for him, which is not necessarily the best for me.'

Despite the initial concerns, shared by Greg's social worker, Norma never considered the possibility that her son would be ill-treated at The Old Rectory. 'It never crossed my mind that they would be anything other than kind to him. I just didn't see that this was a profession that anybody would take up unless they really cared. I was grateful that they were there.'

The decision was made, and Greg moved to The Old Rectory at the end of the school year. It was July, 1981.

Two years later, the Powers were also looking for a residential home. Their social worker told Susan and Davyd she wanted to find the 'right sort of place' for their daughter, somewhere with a 'homely atmosphere' and preferably large grounds to cater for Nicky's love of horses.

'She came along one day and said the home she had in mind was in Somerset, but the people who ran it were now buying a home in Slough and she would like us to go and have a look,' says Susan.

Nicky was by now a sweet-looking teenager, who often carried the slightly disapproving look of a school prefect. She wore a pair of clear-framed glasses and her brown hair brushed forward into a fringe. She visited Stoke Place Mansion House with her parents and saw the horses kept in the grounds. The owner, Gordon Rowe, told Susan and Davyd about the wonderful facilities. They had just opened, so there would be no problem finding her a place, said Rowe.

The Powers found Stoke Place 'shabby' and desperately in need of repairs, with dark and dingy bedrooms and peeling paint. But they were impressed by Rowe's plans for the future. He told them he had only just moved in and would soon be improving the look of the place. Susan thought Gordon was 'a nice man'. 'I thought he was caring. We both thought that,' she says. Susan later discovered that her step-father's first job as a head gardener had been at Stoke Place in the 20s, when it was a grand family home.

A few days before Christmas in 1983, just a month before her seventeenth birthday, Nicky became one of the first residents of Stoke Place. She would not escape for more than ten years.

Rosie

Like Nicky Power, Rosie Valton had been born a healthy baby girl, in Whitechapel, East London. But a brain operation when she was just a few months old left her with a learning difficulty, epilepsy and a partially paralysed right arm. Her mother took her with her when she left England to return to her birthplace of St Lucia two years later. The Caribbean island was to be Rosie's home for the next fourteen years.

When Rosie's mother and grandfather were killed in the great hurricane of 1981, it was left to her grandmother to look after the happy-go-lucky but vulnerable teenager. Caring for Rosie proved too demanding for her, though, and arrangements were made for her to return to London to live with her aunt, Benedict Alcindor.

Benedict had a large family of her own, and within a year realised she would not be able to cope, and would need to find a care home for her niece. She was told of a new home that had opened in Stoke Poges, near Slough. She met the owner, Gordon Rowe, who told Benedict there was a place for her niece at Stoke Place Mansion House. It was January, 1984.

Dorothy

Dorothy Abbott was different from Nicky, Janet, Rosie and the others. She had not been brought up in a loving family environment. Instead, as a little girl, Dorothy had been placed in a series of residential homes, and abandoned by her parents.

Dorothy had cerebral palsy, a condition caused by brain damage. She believes that was the reason her family deserted her. Although she sometimes found it difficult to be understood, she had only a mild learning difficulty. But the 'experts' surmised that if she couldn't talk coherently, then she probably had nothing coherent to say. So Dorothy received practically no education, which only exaggerated her learning difficulties.

In 1963, when Dorothy was about nineteen, she became a resident of Botley's Park long-stay hospital. She was to spend more than twenty years there. Staff brutality was common and conditions harsh. Dorothy remembers sitting down in the huge dining hall for Sunday lunch. 'The patients used to have all the gristle and the stalks of cabbages and the staff used to have the good. A nurse came to me and she said, "You had better eat this or else." I said, "I don't want to eat it." She came back within five minutes, pulled my hair back and tried to stuff it down me.'

Punishments were common if you disobeyed the nursing staff. 'They used to give them bath brush on the feet if they did wrong or give them an injection called 10ccs, or give you a cold bath.' On one occasion, Dorothy and a friend escaped, but were soon picked up by the police. When they were brought back to the hospital, Dorothy spoke up. 'I said, 'You're not going to give me cold bath or you're not going to lock me in a side room or do anything,' and they said no, because I had police witnesses there. They gave me a luke-warm bath, but they didn't give me no bath brush and they tucked me up in a nice warm bed, instead of stripping me in a cold side room.'

By the early 80s, Botley's patients were beginning to be found homes in the community, in preparation for the hospital's eventual closure. The age of the huge, Victorian-style institution was slowly drawing to an end and patients were being resettled in small homes as fast as beds became available.

In December, 1983, Dorothy and her boyfriend, Jimmy, were found places at Stoke Place Mansion House, along with fifteen other Botley's patients.

When Gary Deacon's social worker suggested that Ron should consider Stoke Place, a nearby residential home, he agreed to go and have a look. 'I met Gordon and Angela Rowe and they seemed all right,' says Ron. 'The place seemed OK as well. I agreed reluctantly for him to go there, but it wasn't a nice thing to have to do. I thought that if something happened to me and Gary was still living at home, he could be sent anywhere in the country. At least if he was at Stoke Place he would be nearby for his relatives to visit him.

'I trusted them to look after him. I didn't even consider the possibility that he could be abused. I never thought that anybody in their right mind could take advantage of a mentally handicapped person. With the money they were getting to look after him, I took it that he would be well cared for. I felt very guilty, but I wasn't worried about the place he was going to, just that he was all right. When he first went there, he used to wander around at night looking for me.'

Gary's first visit home was desperately difficult for Ron. 'After he had been there a few weeks, I had him home on a Sunday. Going back to Stoke Place with him at the end of the day was the hardest thing I have ever had to do. We got as far as the Horlicks bridge in Slough [about a mile from Stoke Place] and he started to play up. When we arrived, I had to ask Nigel Rowe [Gordon Rowe's son, who worked at Stoke Place] to help me get Gary out of the car.' On the advice of Gordon Rowe, Ron reluctantly agreed to visit Gary less often, to make it 'easier for him to settle in'.

A couple of years later, Irene Ward discovered, at the age of 46, that she had cancer and had only months to live. She told her husband she had just one remaining wish: to see Janet happily settled in a new home. Her daughter Pauline told me: 'Mum wanted to ensure that she found a permanent home, because she knew my dad couldn't look after her and she didn't want to burden us.'

Janet hated the first home they looked at. Then the family's social worker suggested a large mansion house on the edge of Slough. It was, they were told, set in acres of grounds. Janet would have her own bedroom, instead of a dormitory, and there were classrooms where she could practise her reading and writing.

When Irene, Tony, Pauline and Janet visited Stoke Place, Rowe told them about pub trips, the animals, the swimming pool, the discos, the holidays, all the different activities Janet would enjoy. It sounded too good to be true. Janet loved it.

'We were really impressed with the space and I liked the fact that there was a wide range of abilities and needs,' says Pauline. 'It was a real mixture and she would be able to meet a lot of people her own age.'

'I thought Gordon was lovely and kind. He seemed very fatherly. He said that if a resident wanted to do something they could do it and if they didn't want to they didn't have to. He took me upstairs and showed me the classroom. There were four or five students doing artwork. It was a nice warm environment and there were a lot of colourful paintings on the wall. It just seemed so relaxed. There were all these choices. Mum was absolutely delighted to have found Stoke Place. She thought Janet was going to be very happy there.'

Pauline said her mother also never considered the possibility that Janet would be abused at Stoke Place. 'You did think they might not look after them as well as you looked after them. It's a fact that nobody looks after your children like you do—there was a little bit of that—but never, never did she think of abuse. Apart from that, Janet would have told us. She was vocal. By the time she went to Stoke Place, she could speak properly. The possibility of abuse just didn't occur to us.'

As with the other families that arrived at Stoke Place to meet Gordon Rowe for the first time, the Wards found him charming, if slightly overbearing. He had an answer for every question, a brush-off for every criticism. He left them in no doubt that their children would be cared for, even loved, by him and his staff. Irene returned home reassured and Janet moved to Stoke Place. She was eighteen years old.

Lidia Tunstell was one of the few parents to have reservations about Gordon Rowe. She and Leslie had already visited one home, but its residents were far more able than Stefano and it was completely unsuitable. The social worker suggested Stoke Place. After reading the brochure, the Tunstells visited the home and met manager Desmond Tully, who they found 'charming'. He told them Stefano would have his own room and would work with a small group of residents.

'We said we would talk about it, but the social worker put a lot of pressure on us to send Stefano there,' says Lidia. 'She thought it was good and obviously the fees were much, much cheaper than the fees in Shropshire.

'I put my trust in them. I believed that these people who work with people with disabilities would respect them.'

After a trial run over Easter, Tully phoned Lidia and told her that Stefano was 'very happy' at Stoke Place. Stefano's social worker told them that it seemed to be the right choice. But Lidia didn't like Gordon Rowe and thought his attitude smacked of an 'old time nurse'. 'He wasn't unkind to me and he wasn't rude, but he didn't look like the kind of person to be in charge of young people.' Stefano also seemed 'uneasy', and started to wet himself almost immediately after moving to Stoke Place. But she had little choice. There was a huge shortage of residential places, after all. 'You have to follow the system,' says Lidia. There was always the fear that, if they caused trouble, the local authority would withdraw funding. It is a fear still shared today by nearly every parent of a disabled child.

The decision was made late in 1987, and Stefano became a permanent resident of Stoke Place.

Simon Scott, meanwhile, had been moved from institution to

institution, in search of somewhere able to cope with his particular needs. Finally, his parents were told about Stoke Place.

They drove down to Buckinghamshire from their home in Hornchurch in north-east London one weekend in 1988, and spent the day looking around. They had lunch with Desmond Tully, who told them about the wonderful facilities. He said Simon's epilepsy would not be a problem. Just like so many other parents, they believed Stoke Place would be perfect. At the age of twenty five, they thought, Simon had at last found a permanent home where he would be happy.

Gordon Rowe

10. Broadmoor

> 'I have problems with kids and that stuff. Problems with another case and running away because I am living on my own. I am a tenant. I have had problems throwing snowballs, throwing stones at my windows, throwing snowballs at my front door. For fun, because they want a chase. The police said to me the last time the kids did that to me, they said, 'you're not allowed to hit them or swear at them if you catch them. You could get charged.' It's just where I am staying at the moment. I am hopefully going to be moving in the summer.'
>
> Uisdean Macrae, vice-chair of People First Highlands; 2001

Alfred and Maud Rowe were a well-respected couple in Crowthorne. Alfred, who had fought in the trenches during the First World War, was a railway porter in nearby Camberley. His wife had a reputation for being quiet, calm and hard-working. When she gave birth on September 12, 1934, to the seventh of what were to be ten children, she and Alfred named him Gordon Frank.

When Gordon was six, he began attending Crowthorne Church of England School, a short walk from the family home in the High Street. A former school-mate says he was a fun-loving boy who wasn't particularly bright and 'never showed a serious side to his character'. He had brown hair, in contrast to the ginger hair shared by his four brothers.

The one thing that set Gordon and his siblings apart from their classmates was their love of performing for an audience. If the headmaster, Arthur Goodband, wanted a student to sing to the class or read out a poem, he would often call for a Rowe. Their carol-singing earned their mother money every year to buy them Christmas presents.

The teenage Gordon was an extrovert. He and a friend bought a car, painted it garish colours and slapped on slogans such as 'don't laugh, your daughter might be in here'. He played football for the local Crowthorne Saturday side, as a sturdy and reliable defender. One teammate remembers: 'He showed a lot of team-spirit. I wouldn't say he was ruthless, but he was hard, fair and hard-working. He was a sociable and amicable kind of bloke and I got quite fond of him.'

In Crowthorne there were two options for a school leaver of no exceptional aptitude or intelligence. Either you could join the railways, as two of Gordon's brothers were to do, or you could apply for a job at Broadmoor.

The establishment of the public school Wellington College and the Broadmoor asylum in the latter half of the nineteenth century were the twin reasons Crowthorne had grown from a handful of houses into a small town. Broadmoor was Britain's first Criminal Lunatic Asylum and had been built to take the pressure from the overcrowded Hospital of St Mary of Bethlehem in London. It opened in 1863, was renamed Broadmoor Institution in 1948 and renamed again in 1960, this time as Broadmoor Hospital. But its function remained the same: to hold and treat psychiatric patients of 'dangerous, violent or criminal propensities'.

During the latter half of the 20th century, Broadmoor began to hold a fatal fascination for the media. The tabloids enjoyed nothing better than lurid stories of knife-wielding, escaped 'lunatics' bringing terror to nearby villages.

Despite its rural setting and the beautiful grounds designed for therapeutic effect, Broadmoor retained a reputation for staff brutality. It was also a deeply forbidding place, so much more a prison than a hospital. Its designer, Joshua Jebb, was also responsible for two of the country's most infamous jails—Pentonville and Dartmoor. His Broadmoor squatted on top of a hill, although most of its dark, redbrick buildings were hidden from its neighbours by high perimeter walls.

In the late 50s, Broadmoor was also isolated from the rest of the psychiatric world. There were few reports of its work in specialist journals and it fiercely protected a belief that a strict disciplinarian regime could 'cure' those who passed through its forbidding gates. These patients soon learned that the only way to survive was to conform. If they didn't, they could expect to be beaten black and blue by the 'nurses'.

At the same time, Broadmoor inspired great loyalty and affection. It was common for Crowthorne families to provide staff for generations. Many lived in cosy Victorian cottages on the Broadmoor estate, and found both working and social lives could happily be spent within its boundaries. One Crowthorne resident told me: 'When people went to work up there, you generally never saw them again. Broadmoor was a very close-knit community.'

It was to that community Gordon Rowe applied for a job as a trainee mental health nurse when he returned from national service in the late 50s. One tutor remembers him as a good student: intelligent, alert, caring, and, of course, extrovert. He was said to have got on well with his patients and 'sailed through the course', qualifying as a registered mental nurse in 1962.

'As a student, you could not fault him,' the tutor told me. 'He was a bright lad with a sense of humour. I never heard anything about him which would cause me any disquiet. He was a good lad, and I liked him.'

During the next five years, it is harder to piece together how Rowe's life and career developed. He married in 1962 and left Broadmoor in search of better career opportunities. He and his new wife, Pam, settled in Worcestershire, where he worked with 'mentally handicapped' adults. The council has no record of him now.

In 1967, he moved to Brighton. And it is in Brighton where the story of Gordon Rowe takes its first disturbing turn.

11. Brighton

'In the past few years three of us have been sexually abused... this is on top of discrimination, emotional, and physical abuses we experience all the time... When the three of us were sexually abused, none of us received counselling. We didn't get our rights, even when we went to the police. We just had each other. All of us are still really scared from what happened to us'

Extract from piece written by five members of Milton Keynes People First; *Community Care*; February 13-19, 2003

It was 1974. Rowe was working as a mental health worker for Brighton social services, dealing with mentally ill and 'mentally handicapped' clients. He was certainly well regarded by his superiors, because when a regional ITV documentary team wanted to follow two members of staff, to examine the burdens placed on social workers, Rowe was one of those chosen.

In the film, Rowe portrayed himself as a dedicated professional, struggling to help families on Brighton's deprived housing estates. His approach, he told the camera, was one of 'complete informality'. 'I think when we arrive at a place, we are perhaps treated as a person of authority,' he said. 'I don't like that image. I like to dispense with that image of authority. I like to be considered a friend. One that can be relied upon; one that can be trusted.'

During the documentary, Rowe is seen talking with a learning disabled man of thirty six whose dad has asked for respite care, a truant who won't stop smoking, and a family whose youngest son is running wild. In several scenes, Rowe is seen with a young boy or girl on his lap (a familiarity that would never be permitted in today's social work culture).

But the genial, popular social worker was not all he seemed. Behind the friendly, 'informal' facade lay a darker, disturbing truth.

Evidence that he was sexually assaulting his vulnerable clients was not to be revealed until 1995, when a man contacted police investigating another case. He told them about the social worker who had subjected him to degrading sexual assaults in the back of his car, twenty six years before, when he was nine years old. He described how the man, Gordon Rowe, would drive him to a deserted spot in the country, before having sexual intercourse with him and forcing him to have oral sex in the back seat. He described the car. It was the same vehicle Rowe could be seen driving in the television documentary.

During the documentary, the narrator introduces another of Rowe's visits to his clients: 'The Adams family—Gordon became almost a second father to nine of the sixteen children when Mr Adams went into mental hospital.'

One of the Adams' daughters sits on the arm of the sofa, next to Rowe. Another walks up and sits on his lap, putting her arm around his neck. He places his arm around her waist and continues talking. Angela Adams, one of the sixteen children, was just nine years old when he visited her family for the first time in 1967. More than twenty years later, she was to become his second wife.

As the young girl sits on his lap, Rowe says in voice-over: 'I believe in some of the cases I deal with, I like to think that I am doing some preventative work, not for the immediate future, but perhaps for years to come, with some of the children I'm working with. Maybe I am preventing situations developing with themselves. Perhaps the families that they have will grow up considerably enwisened [sic].'

Whether he had been sexually abusing one of the daughters—one police officer later told me that the investigation team held strong suspicions he had—Rowe had certainly won over Angela's mother. She stared into the camera as she said: 'If it wasn't for Mr Rowe, sometimes I don't know where we would be. Because, I mean, since 1967 when Mr Rowe entered my home, that was the best day's work anybody ever done with us in this family.'

In 1997, Angela was to tell a court that she had not become close to Rowe until he rang her up 'out of the blue' in 1979, and asked her to work for him. Whatever the truth of their relationship, Angela followed him into the care sector after leaving school at sixteen, and worked at a children's centre, an old people's home and a nursery, before taking a year-long residential social work course in 1976 at nearby Lewes Technical College.

By then, Rowe's job had been transferred to East Sussex County Council in the local government shake-up of 1974. Barbara*, a social worker who knew and worked with Rowe in East Sussex, says he 'appeared to care very, very deeply and be very committed to the work he did with the mentally handicapped.

'He was hard-working, diligent, he cared, he had a good rapport with the clients. We would have shopped him if we had known he was abusing anyone.

'We were a fairly tight-knit close group and we all used to meet up. You lived, slept and breathed social services. Gordon Rowe was a larger than life character and he could pull the birds. The only thing I can clearly remember is at a Christmas party. He was loud and over the top and was flirting with all the girls.'

Barbara found Rowe 'quirky' and 'very coarse', but many of his colleagues were, too. 'Social services in Brighton changed dramatically after Maria Colwell [a seven-year-old Brighton girl who was starved, physically abused and killed by her step-father in 1973, under the noses of social services, much like the the murder and child abuse of Victoria Climbié nearly thirty years later which led to a much publicised Public Inquiry], because they then started to recruit from Sussex University. But the old mental welfare officers were a crude lot. They went out to quite horrendous cases when there were not any drugs to use like there are now and they were quite difficult. You are talking about a profession in its infancy.' But, she adds, she would never have described Rowe as a brutal or violent person.

Stuart*, another former colleague, says Rowe was 'very well thought-of by the residents'. 'They loved him. He was very happy-go-lucky, just the type of chap they liked to be around. The first time I met him such a cheer went up as his car pulled up: 'It's Mr Rowe!' He was a bit of an old-fashioned social worker. If he went into somebody's house and a light bulb had blown, he would get on a chair and fix it. He was very down-to-earth and helpful. He would talk to people at their level.'

In 1976, Rowe quit his job. Council records show no evidence of disciplinary problems. Their only existing information comes from his pension records. A spokesman said the absence of any personal files implied there were no 'known concerns' about his behaviour.

However, police officers I have spoken to are convinced he was seeking out and sexually abusing vulnerable people throughout his time in Sussex. He picked his victims well, choosing only those who had no-one to turn to, or could not communicate well. And he used his position of authority to ensure that if anyone did complain, they would not be believed. It was a method he would perfect in future years.

Rowe left the council in 1976 to try for the second time to study for a Certificate of Qualification in Social Work (CQSW). His first attempt had mysteriously ended in failure.

In 1970, Rowe had enrolled on the two-year CQSW course at High Wycombe College of Technology and Art, but withdrew from the course the following June. College records show that he cited 'personal reasons' for quitting. Brighton Council wrote to the college, stating that it would be 'both in the interest of Mr Rowe and also of this Council that he should not return to complete the Social Work course... due to circumstances which are considered to be beyond his control'. Rowe's tutor wrote back to say that he and his colleagues 'fully support Mr Rowe's decision to withdraw as we believe that his personal problems are such that he is unable to reach the required standard either in his academic or in his fieldwork on the course'.

So what were these 'personal problems'? Brighton Council says it has destroyed Rowe's personnel records, so cannot say why he left High Wycombe or why he was allowed to return to work. But one respected social care figure, who was on the High Wycombe course, says Rowe was expelled for cheating in exams and because of 'an issue on one of his practice placements'. Fellow students believed Rowe had had some kind of sexual relationship with a client.

Brighton social services, it seems, was the first in a long string of public authorities that would fail to put an end to Rowe's abuse, and his career in working with vulnerable people. And Rowe was learning how easy it was to avoid detection, and certainly punishment.

In 1976, on leaving East Sussex Council, Rowe tried again for his professional qualification. This time he enrolled at Lewes Technical College. One of his fellow students was Angela Adams, now eighteen years old, who was also taking a social work course at Lewes.

Lewes, since merged with another college, says it no longer has any records relating to Rowe and is unable to comment on whether it knew that Rowe had already had difficulties at a previous college.

After he completed phases I and II of the CQSW at Lewes in 1977, Rowe enrolled at the University of Sussex to finish the qualification. The university says Rowe provided three satisfactory references, including one from East Sussex Council, and there was 'no evidence to suggest that he had been previously excluded from another educational institution'. The following year, he completed his CQSW and returned to Broadmoor, the place that had almost become his spiritual home.

12. From Broadmoor to Somerset

'There appeared to be a culture of silence and non whistle blowing. The conclusion is that a climate was allowed in which a potential abuser would be able to abuse with little chance of quick discovery.'

> Extract from leaked council document with allegations of sexual abuse (unconnected to Gordon Rowe) at a residential home run by Wiltshire County Council; *File on 4*, Radio 4; June 11, 2002

Although Rowe and Pam had now divorced, he obtained married quarters on the Broadmoor estate by telling his superiors that his wife would soon be joining him there.

Ex-colleagues say his second spell at Broadmoor was 'uneasy'. There are tales of him running a pornographic video club at his house every weekend, charging colleagues 50p admission, and of an investigation into the theft of gold rings from a patient.

Broadmoor was essentially the same place Gordon Rowe had left in 1962. There was little therapy, because patients were supposed to be 'treated' through exposure to the rigorous regime. Everyone had to conform, and staff became just as institutionalised as the patients. There were privileges for those who were good, and trips to the 'punishment house' for those who weren't. Patients had to obey to survive.

Much of the daily routine would have been deeply disturbing to outsiders. Inmates were regularly given excessive doses of drugs to sedate them. Plumbing and toilet facilities were poor and there was little for patients to do except the daily routine of cleaning the wards. Beatings were common, but it was a 'golden rule' among nurses that there should be no marks left on the victims, and no witnesses to the attacks. Homosexual relationships between inmates were often tolerated for a time, before staff 'broke them up'. The aim of most patients—many serving long spells for trivial offences—was to stick rigidly to the regime, survive and, hopefully, get out. This was the Broadmoor that Rowe returned to as a social worker. As with his previous spell, it made a great impression on him, and was to provide a blueprint for an institution he would set up for a very different group of clients.

One former colleague says he never suspected that Rowe was not the honest, committed employee he seemed to be. 'Working at Broadmoor could be quite depressing, but he seemed to approach his work in quite a good-natured and amenable way.' He says Rowe was 'at loggerheads' with the psychiatrist in charge of his 'villa' (wing). 'I think Gordon was trying to be more of a social worker, and they weren't regarded in very high esteem. Broadmoor was seen as more of a prison than a hospital and Gordon wanted to rehabilitate people. He came across as someone who was relaxed, rather than as a tough disciplinarian. But he probably conned me as well, because he knew I had different views from the establishment.'

Within a few months, Rowe began telling colleagues he planned to leave and open a residential home for 'mentally handicapped' people. Many other Broadmoor staff were doing the same thing. There was an enormous shortage of residential and nursing beds around the country, and the Conservative government of Margaret Thatcher, in its desire to stimulate the private sector, would soon introduce legislation to allow entrepreneurs to set up care homes, unhindered by red tape. Although the move would increase the supply of such homes, many of them were owned by business people intent on cutting corners wherever they found them. There was a lot of money to be made if the homes were big enough and the running costs kept low enough. Mrs Thatcher's policy created an avalanche of new homes but at the cost of turning learning disabled people into a commodity. Such a culture was bound to expose many people with learning difficulties to poor standards of care and the risk of neglect and abuse.

In 1980, Rowe heard from a friend about an ideal property. The small hotel in west Somerset, formerly the village rectory, had been put up for sale by its businessman owner, David Fineberg. Rowe told Fineberg he had money to invest in a residential home. Fineberg met Rowe and was impressed by his enthusiasm, and agreed to apply for planning permission to convert the hotel into a home for 20 'mentally handicapped' adults.

But residents of West Quantoxhead were horrified at the idea of 'mentally ill' patients living at The Old Rectory. They called a protest meeting and talked of the risk of 'dangerous' undesirables terrorising girls at the village school. But Rowe's apparent sincerity in wishing to create a caring environment won over the local council. Permission was granted and the home opened.

Within weeks, the venture ran into problems. Rowe admitted to Fineberg that he had no money to invest. His financial backers probably never existed. Fineberg thought about pulling out, but Rowe convinced him the project would be enormously profitable, so he financed the home himself and made Rowe his care director.

Fineberg, now still running The Old Rectory and another Somerset home, told me: 'He was a very plausible person, in the same way that a con-man is a plausible person.'

Gordon Rowe hadn't come to Somerset alone. His assistant was Angela Adams, who he had brought with him from Brighton. They shared a two-bedroom flat at The Old Rectory with Rowe's son, Nigel, and five large dogs.

The residents appeared to worship their care director. 'They all seemed to love him and called him "dad"', says one friend. 'I thought the guy was magic.' He was not the only one. In 1982, a reporter from the *West Somerset Free Press* visited The Old Rectory and compiled a glowing feature about the work of the—as the article mistakenly described him—'burly Londoner'.

Rowe told him: 'What I set out to do, and what I think we are achieving, is giving these kids a place to grow up which they regard as home rather than an institution. Once here, they tend to grow up rapidly, as they realise they are no longer living in a children's world.'

He told the journalist how several of the mainly young men had developed 'almost miraculously' in their short time at the home. 'Aggressive behaviour is not tolerated. If they do try this sort of thing when they first come here, they soon learn it is better to behave properly. Anyone who looks likely to upset the rapport we have established or cause trouble is sent back on the next train.'

Rowe came across, as he would many times over the next decade, as a tough but caring professional, intent on providing a loving environment.

13. Like a Zombie

'Abuse against vulnerable people may not come to light and if it does is unlikely to be reported to the police. There are considerable difficulties in both investigation and prosecution and because of evidential difficulties cases may not proceed to court.'

Home Office consultation paper,
Setting the Boundaries, Reforming the Law on Sex Offences, July 2000

For the first eighteen months, Norma Adams thought everything at The

Old Rectory was fine. For the first six months, Rowe had asked her not to visit her son, to give him time to 'settle in'. Reluctantly, she had agreed, but as Greg could not speak, she couldn't telephone him, either.

Greg seemed to settle in well, though, and the family visited regularly during 1982. But by the early months of 1983, Norma and Greg's social worker both began to question Rowe's failure to set up therapy sessions or expand the range of activities. Norma later discovered that most residents spent all day chopping wood or working in the gardens.

Norma arrived for one visit to find Greg 'like a zombie'. He had been heavily and inappropriately dosed with Largactil, a drug used to treat symptoms of psychosis. (The drug is commonly used inappropriately for learning disabled people.) Soon afterwards, she received a call from Carol Smith*, who lived nearby and had taken a keen interest in the home. She had seen Greg wandering down the main road and believed the residents were being neglected and that some of the more capable men were being exploited.

In fact, Carol and her husband David got on well with Rowe. David Smith found him 'an overtly friendly type of robust person' and was impressed by his 'great air of enthusiasm and optimism'. He believed Rowe when he said all he needed was enough money to carry out the changes he wanted to make. 'He really gave the impression that he wanted it to be nice for them, to make a new life for people who came from difficult backgrounds.' He twice took up invitations to inspect The Old Rectory, and was even asked to invest in a home Rowe was planning to open in Bucks. Astonishingly, Rowe gave the Smiths a list of local authorities with clients at The Old Rectory, so they could write to complain about the home.

'Rowe told me it was very difficult for him, because he didn't have enough money to run the place properly,' Carol told me. 'He said his own home would be nothing like this one.' On another occasion, he told the couple he was taking eight of the 'boys' on a free holiday, but hadn't been given any money to buy them treats.

The Smiths blamed other staff for the problems, and wrote to Somerset social services, complaining about the standard of care. They said they had frequently seen residents running around outside in slippers and unsuitable clothes, and residents would often go missing in the nearby Quantock Hills. The Smiths had been convinced by Rowe's air of vigorous affability and thought him blameless, even though he was running the home. They were merely the latest to join the long line of those who were to be taken in.

Norma Adams also complained to Somerset social services, as well as Avon and Somerset Police, the charity Mencap, and Greg's social worker. 'I had serious concerns about the standards of care and I thought Greg was having much too heavy doses of tranquillisers,' she says. She believes the resulting enquiries were 'superficial'. A spokeswoman for the London Borough of Hammersmith and Fulham says the council was unable to trace the relevant records.

Chris Davies, who was responsible for children's services in 1983 and is now director of Somerset social services, told me he had been through the files 'with a fine toothed comb'. He says the only complaints received were 'general management issues and in particular around the impact on the neighbourhood of behaviour in the home'.

Meanwhile, Fineberg's relationship with Rowe was deteriorating. He suspected him of dishonesty, and noted his habit of drawing bundles of crisp bank-notes from his pockets. He describes him as 'behaving like Julius Caesar, some sort of emperor, but with sinister overtones'. Eventually, he discovered Rowe had held an open day for the residential home he was setting up in Buckinghamshire, and planned to take as many residents with him as he could. Fineberg confronted him, took legal advice and Rowe agreed to go.

Fineberg then asked Michael Brown*, a former colleague of one of his employees, to take over. But Rowe was not yet ready to open his home and wanted to stay on for a few more weeks. It took a meeting with the chairman of the local Mencap group for him to agree to leave.

Brown remembers the meeting. 'It was a very strange and bizarre situation to walk into and, although Gordon accepted he would abide by his decision to leave, he remained full of antipathy about his relationship with Fineberg. Rowe saw himself as all-important, a patriarchal figure. He told me: "I am there when they get up in the morning, and I am there when they go to bed in the evening." He was a very bombastic guy.' Rowe eventually left in late July.

Rowe's departure was not universally welcomed. Many of the social workers with clients at the home were unhappy at the way he had been treated. Fineberg believed they liked his 'lack of polish'. And, after all, he was one of them.

When Rowe finally left, he took four residents, a lot of personal possessions belonging to those who stayed behind, and presents bought for them with the proceeds of a charity bed race. He was joined by various members of staff, including Angela Adams, Nigel Rowe and a bespectacled, teenaged care assistant called Desmond Tully. Tully had borrowed £8,000 from his bank and lent it to Rowe to help him start his business.

At the time they left, there was only one qualified employee in the home. Rowe had taken on mostly untrained and unqualified boys and girls, filling their heads with techniques and theories he had picked up during his time at Broadmoor. It was a method he was to repeat in Buckinghamshire.

Fineberg remembers driving to the home and watching Rowe load up a removal lorry. 'Anything that wasn't nailed down disappeared with him.'

Fineberg went about recruiting new staff, and for the first time the home was being run by experienced care workers.

It seems to have taken only a few days after Rowe's departure for Albert*, a thirty-four-year-old resident from Brent, to confide in a member of staff that Rowe had been sexually assaulting him. The allegation was passed on to Brown and Fineberg, who contacted Mike Furlong, Somerset's registration and inspection officer. Furlong said the allegations would have to be investigated by the police, not by the council.

'If it were now, we would almost certainly have done the investigation jointly with the police,' Chris Davies told me later. 'But at that time, we handed it to the police to do themselves. There was no suggestion that it was anybody other than Rowe, so there was no issue about the current protection of those people.'

At about this time, clinical psychologist Madeleine Thomas visited The Old Rectory to assess Albert. She had been there before, but had turned down Rowe's offer of work because she didn't trust him. 'Something about him made me feel he wasn't honest. I also didn't like the way he treated the residents. I thought he was rather autocratic,' she says.

The interview confirmed her fears. Albert appeared frightened and upset, and told her how Rowe had made him visit his flat four times a week for mutual masturbation. He had no idea that what Rowe was doing was wrong. Rowe had threatened to send him back to the long-stay hospital he had come from if he told anybody what he was doing. He also gave him 'special privileges'.

Appalled—especially when she discovered Rowe was setting up his own home—Thomas, now head of department for a Somerset hospital trust, informed Fineberg and rang Somerset social services. During her career, she has given evidence in court many times as an expert witness and believes Albert provided a number of details he could not have made up.

Two detectives interviewed Albert and at least one other resident. On October 3, they travelled to Buckinghamshire to interview Rowe about allegations of gross indecency. There was no solicitor, but Angela Adams, introduced as Gordon's common-law wife, insisted on being present. Rowe was quizzed thoroughly, but told the officers nothing to corroborate the allegations. They passed a report to their detective chief inspector. He decided that no charges could be brought, so the inquiry was closed and Somerset social services were briefed. They notified Bucks County Council, as did one of the police officers.

The two officers were so upset at their failure to secure a prosecution that they returned to The Old Rectory with armfuls of presents for the residents. They told staff they believed Gordon Rowe was guilty, but just couldn't prove it.

When Fineberg realised that, despite Albert's courage in revealing how he had been abused, there wasn't going to be a trial, he contacted Buckinghamshire County Council to warn them about Rowe, even though the authorities in Somerset told him they would do this themselves. 'I was convinced Rowe's registration in Bucks would not be confirmed,' he told me.

Over the next few weeks, staff at The Old Rectory talked to every one of the residents about Rowe. 'There were other young men and women who were not able to give an intelligible account of what had happened to them,' says Brown. 'One of them demonstrated what Rowe had done to him with a mime and said, 'he do that, he do that'. We eventually decided there were about 15 residents who had been abused. There was no corroborating evidence, but none of the staff were in any doubt. We all knew these things had happened. Unfortunately, short of getting them into the witness box, there was nothing that could be done. Even if they had gone into the witness box, Rowe had a tremendous amount of power over the residents and he would have employed that to intimidate them in court.'

Brown wrote at the end of November to a resident's social worker in Kent. He also contacted Bucks County Council. The registration department told him there was nothing they could do if the allegations were not proven. He says they inferred that he—who had only met Gordon Rowe twice—was motivated by malice. He believes they were told to expect his call.

Brown says Rowe ran the home as a 'punitive regime', with residents given privileges which could be removed if they misbehaved. The home was 'a custodial place for people who had to be punished and it was Gordon Rowe's God-given right to punish them'. One male resident took a cake from the bread van and was sent to his bedroom for six weeks as a punishment.

Brown, Fineberg, Thomas, Norma Adams and the Smiths were not the only ones raising concerns about The Old Rectory. When Brent social services heard of the allegations, they wrote to Somerset, prodded by Albert's social worker. Six months later, following an exchange of letters with Somerset social services, Brent wrote to the Department of Health and Social Security, expressing concern about the case. They also spoke to Buckinghamshire social services. Again, nothing was done.

Today, Albert lives in a hospital. Because of the abuse he suffered at the hands of Gordon Rowe, and the effect it has had on his own behaviour, he is incapable of living in the community. Although he has only moderate learning difficulties, he is likely to spend the rest of his life in an institution.

14. Sensitive, Able and Caring

> 'Social work chiefs are being forced to find inventive ways to cope with crippling staff shortages… according to a study commissioned by Community Care magazine. Many local authorities in London had between 25 and 40 per cent vacancy rates for social workers, rising to 80 per cent in some individual teams'
>
> *The Independent*, June 18, 2002

Rowe had picked another struggling hotel as the location for his own residential home.

Stoke Place Mansion House in Stoke Poges, on the edge of Slough, had been bought as an investment by South Bucks District Council in the 60s, together with two hundred acres of surrounding land, and turned into a nursing home. After a fire, a funeral director took it on at a peppercorn rent, repaired the damage and converted it into a country club. In 1978, he sold the lease to David George and his wife Chris, and two business partners.

The Georges turned Stoke Place into a two-star hotel. After initially thriving, the recession bit, and by the early 80s they were desperate for a new business partner. For Rowe, the location was ideal, near London and its plentiful supply of potential clients, and only 25 minutes drive from Crowthorne, where he was born.

Rowe was introduced to David George through a mutual friend. George was impressed. 'He could make one feel very emotional about the mentally handicapped and the lot they had,' he told me.

Rowe even talked about his relationship with Fineberg and confessed to taping their conversations. 'There were lots of little things like that which should have warned me not to get involved. One should have twigged that he was a bit strange,' said George. But their discussions progressed well and they agreed to split Stoke Place into two, with the Georges running a country club in one half and Rowe setting up a residential home in the other.

'Gordon hadn't any money and we hadn't any money,' says Chris George. 'We got a joint short-term bank loan to do up the property. The council would not let us have the head lease and sub-let to Gordon, so we were co-lessees. It was sink or swim. Without them, we would have lost here and lost our house. At that stage, they saved us.'

Another businessman who helped Rowe launch his company was car-dealer Raymond Beck. Already past retirement age, Beck had been approached by his accountant, who also acted for Rowe, to ask whether he wished to invest. Beck agreed. 'They apparently had to pay a sum up front for the tenancy and there was a shortfall,' he says. 'My accountant asked if I was interested and I said yes.' He paid £23,500 for a quarter share in the business. Rowe bought the shares back the following July and gave them to Nigel, but Beck says he made no profit. 'It was all done as a sort of charity,' he told me.

London solicitor Geoffrey Preston, who became the company secretary and advised Rowe on setting up Longcare Ltd—the company which would run the home—visited Stoke Place and was impressed by Rowe's plans. Preston, also briefly a Longcare company director, says: 'He seemed confident it would work and, what was more important, he convinced other people it would work. He didn't strike me as being anything out of the ordinary, apart from somebody who was really quite impressive in being able to put together something like that.' Preston parted company with Longcare in the late 80s when Rowe moved to a cheaper legal adviser.

Before Rowe could apply to have his home registered by Bucks social services, he needed the permission of South Bucks District Council, which owned the building, to convert the Mansion House from a hotel to a care home. The letter he wrote was perfectly pitched to appeal to local councillors—it talked about the jobs the new business would create, the educational benefits for the residents and the 'family' atmosphere Rowe would bring with him from Somerset. It was persuasive, reassuring, down-to-earth and tugged gently at the heart-strings. No-one reading it would have had the slightest idea about the frightening regime of sexual abuse over which Rowe had presided at The Old Rectory.

He told the council that none of the residents would have 'any previous history or record of aggression or anti-social behaviour' or 'sexual deviance'. Most of them, he said, had come from long-stay hospitals. He stressed the 'family life' The Old Rectory had offered, which would be replicated at Stoke Place, supplemented by educational and social training, such as trips to the cinema, Windsor Castle, and David George's country club.

Rowe talked about the 'very able working lads' at The Old Rectory in Somerset, who had worked in the kitchen gardens, cleared the woods and grounds of brambles, and cut logs for the fire. And he described the 'special projects' they had taken on, such as tidying old people's gardens, picking fruit, and maintaining the 20-mile length of the West Somerset Steam Railway track. At Stoke Place, the working lads would help to clear the lake, the kitchen gardens and the woods.

All the residents, he said, 'have their own individual personalities, their likes and dislikes, their fears, hopes and aspirations'. Many would come from London, so Stoke Place would be ideally suited for visits from relatives. 'Contact of this nature is seen by us as essential to developing the individual and to help him reach his maximum potential,' he added.

'I could go on with the benefits for us, for the Stoke Place Country Club and for the surrounding community,' he wrote, 'but this may become boring and be misconstrued as an attempt at overselling ourselves, rather than an attempted straightforward and honest description of how I see the future and how we can complement each other.'

It was a fantastically crafted letter—but it was anything but straightforward and honest.

Some councillors were still sceptical that a country club and a residential home could exist as neighbours. But Rowe knew exactly how to appeal to their sympathies and emotions when he spoke at a council committee meeting in 1983. He spoke eloquently about the environment he would create, and the care he would provide for some of the most needy people in society. He quoted government reports and care experts and produced references and the cutting from the Somerset newspaper. The councillors were also impressed to read a letter from Rowe's banker, which stated that the home was potentially very profitable.

A possible hitch was the copy of the report from Somerset police, which had landed on the desk of council solicitor Tony Levings. He questioned Rowe, but was fed the story of sour grapes and unfounded allegations. The district councillors voted to grant Rowe permission to convert part of the Mansion House into a care home.

The final and highest hurdle was to have the home registered with Bucks County Council. For that to happen, its registration department would have to view Rowe as a suitable person to be looking after 'mentally handicapped' people.

Bucks County Council has never accepted it failed to make proper checks on Rowe's background. A spokesman told me they received good references, as well as a 'communication' from Fineberg. But they admitted that a reference from Somerset County Council, describing Rowe as 'a sensitive, able and caring man' with a 'good understanding of the needs of those mentally handicapped people placed within his care, together with a keen interest in their welfare', was written six months before the allegations investigated by Somerset CID came to light.

The council admits none of its staff visited Somerset to check on the allegations. Public relations chief Bob Bird said in 1996: 'At that time, the registration procedure focussed mainly on the qualifications of the people running homes and the suitability and safety of the buildings. Mr Rowe, himself, told us about the allegations made by the owner of another private residential home in Somerset, and about which Buckingham social services was, in fact, already aware. These allegations were discussed with Somerset social services and Somerset police, who told us they had been investigated and that the file had been closed after a thorough investigation.'

Chris Davies says his staff phoned Bucks to tell them about the police inquiry and its outcome. 'Everybody felt pretty uneasy and people at the home felt he might have abused more widely. Mike Furlong was not in a position to have said that (Rowe was guilty) himself, but he would not have disagreed with that. Bucks were aware that, while no criminal charges were brought, there was not exactly a clean bill of health. In those days that was a very common position to end up in, because of judicial views about the quality of evidence people with learning disabilities can give. It would have been a guarded message, as they often are, which would have said, "that was the criminal finding, but that ain't the whole story".

Davies admits his council was conned by Gordon Rowe. 'Almost everyone who dealt with Gordon Rowe in Somerset thought he was absolutely wonderful. [If you had tried to take action against him] you would have had any number of statements from families, from agencies, saying this guy is absolutely tremendous. There is no doubt that he took us in.'

Bucks County Council received four references for Rowe, all of which had also been used with his planning application. Two were from professionals who had provided David George with glowing tributes a year earlier. Ieuan Williams, chief education officer at Broadmoor, had known Rowe for 20 years. He described his departure from Broadmoor as 'a great loss' and said he had been 'regarded with great esteem' by his colleagues and 'was popular and well liked' by patients. He said he was 'absolutely trustworthy, sincere and loyal'. Williams described The Old Rectory as 'a therapeutic environment' and said Rowe was 'idolized by the boys and girls who are resident there'.

A second reference was written by Richard Holley, who described Rowe's 'unique rapport with mentally handicapped people' and his 'natural flair' for social work. Holley was a senior officer in Kensington and Chelsea's mental health section. He had found places at The Old Rectory for two men who had been living in hospitals for 30 years. When he visited them, he remembers being impressed with the ease with which Rowe dealt with 'potentially explosive' situations. 'I remember one occasion after dinner in the evening, and two of the fellows got a bit excited, and one of them really clobbered the other one in the face. Gordon Rowe took one of them to the side and said to him: 'You must not do that. Say sorry to him.' Then he took him upstairs. I thought that was pretty good, that he had defused it straight away. It stuck in my mind, someone knowing what to do in awkward circumstances, because the one who had been slapped around the face was quite distressed.

'My lads were always happy when I saw them. They never had anything to say against Gordon Rowe, even when he wasn't there.'

The other two references were from Furlong and a Somerset fire officer. There was no reference from David Fineberg, and none requested by Bucks.

Despite the concerns of Madeleine Thomas, David Fineberg, Michael Brown, Somerset County Council, and the police investigation, Rowe was home and dry. Members of Bucks County Council went along with the advice of their officers. They believed Rowe was a fit person to be running a residential home for vulnerable adults.

On November 28, 1983, Gordon Rowe was registered by Bucks County Council to care for thirty eight 'mentally handicapped' adults at Stoke Place Mansion House.

LONGCARE

15. Welcome to Stoke Place

> 'A teenager who carried out a vicious attack on a vulnerable family in their home had his sentence reduced to 18 months yesterday... they forced the father to eat human faeces and compelled both him and his wife to perform oral sex 'under the threat of killing the father if they did not'... The gang also threatened to cut off the father's penis... The court had been told that the three had targeted the family 'for a laugh' because they knew the parents had learning difficulties.'
>
> The Independent, February 16, 2002

1999

Dorothy Thomson (née Abbott) is sitting in an armchair in the cosy flat in a small town in the south of England she shares with her husband, Jamie. It is nearly nine years since she left Stoke Place. She wears a bright green woollen sweater. Her glasses have thick lenses and her grey hair is tied back in a ponytail. Dorothy's fingers are stiff and twisted by cerebral palsy and her movements are jerky. Her voice occasionally quavers when she emphasises a point. The years she has spent in institutions and her lack of a formal education are betrayed by the occasional slightly inappropriate use of an unfamiliar word.

DOROTHY: I had a social worker and he took the other residents up to

Stoke Place and they would come back and say how great it was

JP: *How many people went to Stoke Place from Botley's Park?*

DOROTHY: There was quite a few. I had to have a fight to get there because I was still with this boyfriend of mine, Jimmy [not her present husband]. 'Cos Gordon Rowe said, 'I only want one,' but then the social worker said, 'You will have to take them both, because they are both mates to each other.' So we ended up there, but I never knew...

1983

In the beginning there were just a few residents at Stoke Place Mansion House. Some came with Gordon Rowe from Somerset, late in 1983. Over the next nine months, another 17 men and women, including Dorothy and Jimmy, arrived from Botley's Park. Hospitals like Botley's were desperate to find beds, as they began to return patients to the community. Residential home bosses like Rowe were only too happy to take them in.

After sleeping for years in dormitory wards where their only possessions were kept in little wooden lockers by their beds, it would have been natural for them to be overwhelmed by Stoke Place, a beautiful home in the country, with a lake and farm animals, and their own bedrooms. They must have felt grateful to Rowe for bringing them there.

16. Red Apples, Green Apples

'Thousands of disabled children who have been abused are falling through cracks in the child protection system, campaigners have claimed. A new National Working Group on Child Protection and Disability, which includes major charities, is to call on the government to urgently fund research into the issue. This comes as the jailing of a special needs teacher has again revealed the vulnerability of children with disabilities. A jury at Newcastle Crown Court heard how Malcolm Phillips, aged fifty one, of Mowbray Close, Sunderland, choked autistic children at a residential school and stood on their faces and hair.'

Disability Now, January 2002

1999

DOROTHY: *I must say Gordon Rowe was a very, very dominating man.*

He didn't like anybody not liking him. He liked every resident to like him. He also didn't like you if you was intelligent on making things and if you could read, or if you could do writing of any description. He hated that. I think that he was a man that always wanted to be in the limelight.

1988

Debbie* had only been at Longcare for a few months, but she was one of the better-qualified staff. At first, she had thought Longcare was wonderful. 'You were shown around and shown the best of everything,' she would say later. 'You read the prospectus and it sounded like a wonderful holiday camp. Until you actually got to work there.'

She worked at Stoke Green, the second Longcare home, across the road from Stoke Place. Most staff felt Stoke Green was a more relaxed place to work, but it only took a few months for Debbie to become disturbed by some of the things she was witnessing. Although she needed the money, the stress of working there was making her ill.

The young man leaned forward, looked at the bus and screwed up his eyes. He looked up at Debbie, who was sat opposite him, behind her desk in the Stoke Green office. He smiled. 'Blue?' he asked.

'No, it's red. London buses are red. Let's try another one.' She turned the page of the book and pointed to an apple.

John F smiled again. 'Apple, Debbie. Apples is red. Red, Debbie?' John was taller and stronger than most of the other residents. He was one of Gordon's favourites and helped with the security at Stoke Place. But he also acted as a spy. He kept an eye on residents and staff and reported back to Gordon. When he saw a care assistant give a resident an extra cup of tea, he reported it. He was given special privileges in return. John was capable of living independently, but it suited Gordon to keep him at Longcare, and away from the classroom.

'Some apples are red, but this one's green,' said Debbie.

'You're wasting your bloody time.'

Debbie looked up. 'You're wasting your time. He'll never learn colours.' Gordon Rowe stood in front of the desk.

'If I can teach him colours, John can get work as a painter. He's so artistic, and you know how hard he works.'

'I told you. You're wasting your time. I don't want you doing this anymore. John, no more colours,' said Rowe. He slammed his hand down on the open book.

'Yes, Gordon,' said John, and nodded fast, twice, as Rowe turned for

the door. Debbie, her face flushed, followed him. He swivelled round, standing so close they were nearly toe-to-toe.

Debbie took a step back. 'Gordon, he's talented enough to work for a living as a decorator.' She noticed Rowe was flushed and trembling.

'I don't want you helping him,' he repeated, and marched out, slamming the door behind him.

Later that week, John was moved across the road to Stoke Place, away from Debbie and Stoke Green.

Rowe's need to control and dominate the residents he cared for extended far beyond their education and what he called their 'social training'. He was only content if he was ruling every aspect of their lives.

He ordered staff to inform him of all instances of 'sexual activity', even if it was only a kiss on the cheek, and he kept track of which residents were going out together. If he didn't like a pairing, he would split them up and tell the two residents who to go out with instead.

It was just one of the many ways in which Gordon Rowe imposed his will on his clients. Choosing your own friends was a simple right taken for granted outside the high walls of Longcare, but one that Rowe pilfered, and wrenched out of shape.

To his staff, many of whom were young and inexperienced, his words made a kind of sense. After all, he was a trained social worker. Surely he knew what he was doing. And, as he told his employees, he had been in the social care field for nearly thirty years.

Rowe had developed a range of punishments to help him control the residents. Anyone who was 'naughty'—those who disobeyed his orders—might be locked in their room for days on end, or have their pocket money (from their own social security allowance) confiscated. Those who were late for meals, even by only a few seconds, were not allowed to eat.

They were the kind of punishments that, in a much less exaggerated form, might have been appropriate for an eight-year-old child who had been rude to her parents. But these were adults.

Rowe treated the residents as naughty kids. It allowed him to control and restrict their independence to a far greater extent than if he had dealt with them as adults. But he could easily justify it to his care assistants. He would explain that a man with the reasoning powers of an eight-year-old child should be treated—and punished—like an eight-year-old child. 'It's the only way they learn,' he would say. His young, unskilled employees could only nod their heads and carry on with their work.

17. Lottie Perfume

> 'It was common ground between the various witnesses that in about early 1997 water pistols were brought into the Home and were used by care staff and residents in play. However, we find that over time they also came to be used in particular on resident A to keep him awake in the early evening so that he would not wake in the night and disturb staff and other residents. DT raised the matter with JH who told him it was alright as care staff needed a good night's sleep.'
>
> Extract from Registered Homes Tribunal case concerning a home for adults with learning disabilities; heard on various dates between January and May, 2000

1999
DOROTHY: Gordon played with our feelings so much, me and Jimmy. He tried to actually send me mental. I was so strong that I wouldn't get it.

What kept me from going mental, once you went to those places you've got to be full of hate and you have to have a dream to cling onto. My dream seemed impossible to me. My dream was that, one day, I would be free, I would have my own flat, I would settle down, and I never let go of that dream.

1990
Gordon loved to make fun of the residents. He thought there was nothing funnier than mocking *Tim*, who was very effeminate, about buying ladies' jewellery. And he loved humiliating *Peter*, who would come downstairs in the middle of the night and masturbate on the sofa. Rowe would shout at him in front of other residents, calling him 'a dirty bastard'. Peter would sit there, his head sunk into his chest, two fingers tapping his nose, as he rocked backwards and forwards.

'Gordon would stand behind Tony, who was blind, and make him jump,' one staff member recalls. 'He mocked Tim all the time and made him dress up in girls' clothes. He also took the mickey out of staff behind their backs, so the clients could have a laugh.'

Another member of staff remembers Rowe lying in wait for Peter, who was also blind, as he walked down the stairs at Stoke Place. As Peter reached the bottom, Rowe shouted at him, and then tripped him up when he jumped in shock. He then sauntered back to his office, chuckling.

Lottie, who was incontinent, was another who became the butt of Gordon Rowe's 'jokes'. Whenever a resident was incontinent, he would shout: 'Smells like someone's got their Lottie perfume on.' Some learning disabled people find bowel and bladder control a problem, especially after epileptic seizures.

In this way, Rowe taught the staff not to respect the residents, and vice versa. This made it less likely that residents would trust the care workers, and less likely that they would care enough about residents to object to their ill-treatment.

An outsider who witnessed one of these incidents might have put Rowe's behaviour down to a childish love of pranks. But Rowe was steadily redrawing the boundaries for his staff on what was acceptable. By displaying such behaviour, he set an example as well as the standard for Longcare. The more he mocked and humiliated the residents, the less likely it became that a care worker would risk their job and object, if Rowe stepped even further over the boundary.

None of the residents would have been surprised to be humiliated in this way. Learning disabled people learn to expect nothing better. It's only a short step from viewing someone as inferior to turning a blind eye to a kick, a slap, or a punch.

18. Gordon's Listening

> 'Social isolation remains a problem for people with learning disabilities. A recent study (Hester Adrian Research Centre, University of Manchester, 1999) found that only 30 per cent had a friend who was not either learning disabled or part of their family or paid to care for them.'
>
> *Valuing People: A New Strategy for Learning Disability for the 21st Century*, Department of Health White Paper, March 2001

1999
DOROTHY: *The boys like John F and John M, they were the spies to look*

out for places. Gordon Rowe wanted to get me like that. He said, 'I'll leave you in here. Keep an eye on the residents. Don't let them go to sleep, don't let them leave the room.' But I would let them go to sleep and John M would say, 'he's going to sleep, you better got to wake them up.' But I said, 'No, I'm not. He's allowed to go to sleep. I'm not going to wake him up.' But then I didn't know that it was John M would go back to Gordon Rowe and tell Gordon Rowe that I let the residents sleep through the day.

1991
Clare Johnson remembers how Rowe had described Stoke Place as some sort of glorious rural paradise, more holiday park than residential home, when she came for her interview, aged eighteen. She enjoyed working with the residents, even the ones with behavioural problems, but the first few weeks had not been easy. She had already started to wonder about the way her boss treated some of the residents: the slaps, the dirty jokes, the mickey-taking. But she was young and inexperienced. What did she know? After all, they called him Big Dada. Maybe he was just playing the part of a strict, loving father.

She put the video camera back on her shoulder and tried to hold it steady as she gave the piece of string to Joyce with her other hand. Threading beads. That was all Joyce had been doing for years. She was blind, and Rowe had told Clare she was unable to do anything more difficult.

Clare followed Joyce as she prepared the string for the next bead. She swept the video camera across the classroom in a slow arc, catching the other men and women as they worked. Some drew on cheap pieces of paper, others looked at pictures in magazines.

Clare was filming the class as part of a project for her college course in care work. Gordon had shown her the video-editing suite in his cottage in the grounds of Stoke Place. It was full of gadgets and rows of labelled tapes. He explained how the different machines worked, but she hadn't taken much of it in. She had been delighted when he offered to edit her video. Her mum, an experienced care worker herself, was impressed with Gordon's interest.

Clare walked across the classroom. One resident sat and stared at a pile of coloured plastic rings, another fiddled with a felt-tip pen and a third flicked listlessly through a clothes catalogue. She walked back between the tables and turned the camera to the rest of the class as they plucked slowly at their tasks. The door opened behind her and she saw Gordon's stocky figure enter the frame. She followed him with the camera as he headed towards the table where Michael sat drawing.

Gordon waved her away. 'I think Jackie needs some help, Clare,' he said.

As she turned again and walked back towards the other end of the room, she heard a crack.

She swivelled the camera back towards Gordon. She saw Michael cowering in his seat, Gordon standing over him.

The bell sounded.

As the residents left the room, Gordon called Clare to him. 'Just about finished now, is it?' he said.

She fiddled with the camera as she walked towards him, unable to look him in the eye. She pretended to examine the eject button. 'Yes, I think so.'

'Well, give me a week or so, and I'll have it ready. Save you all the bother with the cutting and the editing.' And he held out his hand.

She hesitated, but only for a couple of seconds. She pressed the eject button on the camera. 'Thanks, Gordon,' she said.

Susannah* was another care assistant who had been impressed by Rowe at her job interview. 'He interviewed me in reception. He even asked my husband to sit in, and he was giving us so much spiel about how fantastic it was and how the clients went off to America for holidays. He never showed me round. I did ask, but he said he was a little bit busy at the moment. I had never worked with people with learning disabilities, only with the elderly and children, so I thought it was a bit strange that he gave me the job. But I thought he was fantastic, very caring, very polite, and the way he was talking was that the things the clients had were absolutely out of this world.'

Susannah soon found out that the reality of working at Longcare didn't match up to Gordon's public relations. 'My first day, one of the male clients had an outburst and smashed some cups. It frightened me a bit. He was led out by Gordon Rowe, and he gave him a clunk round the head. Gordon saw that I was shocked and said, 'That's how you have to deal with them.' But I said, 'I wouldn't treat my dog like that.' I don't know what made me do it, but I went back to work the next day.'

Rowe used as many young and inexperienced staff as he could. They were much easier to intimidate, and were paid very low wages. Many came on Youth Training Schemes. If any of his employees dared question his behaviour, he warned them that he could make sure they never worked in the care industry again. Most of them had never seen the inside of a residential home before, or met anyone with a learning difficulty, so they generally did as they were told.

Not all of the staff were wet behind the ears, though. Some had worked in residential care before, but that didn't mean they knew how to cope with a boss like Gordon Rowe. Few of them had any professional qualifications and they were isolated and intimidated. Rowe made sure it stayed that way: he was the boss, and those who didn't agree with what he told them could find another job. The residents, of course, did not have that option.

Rowe seemed to detect potential trouble instinctively, and knew when to apply pressure on his staff. He also knew his care assistants, many of whom were young and inexperienced, would not stand up to him. But there were far more sinister techniques he used to maintain order.

Rowe spied on everyone. Not just with the video camera he carried around, but also by listening to the conversations of residents and staff. He had an intercom installed so he could listen in to rooms all over Stoke Place, just by pressing a button on the control box. The care workers found out and started to communicate using Makaton—the sign language designed for people with learning difficulties—until Rowe saw them and banned it.

Rowe often used spurious, but persuasive, explanations for such decisions. On this occasion, he told staff that using Makaton would 'embarrass parents seeing their daughter or son signing to them while they were walking down the high street'. With his charisma and powers of persuasion, he was usually able to convince his staff that he was right.

Those who weren't convinced were too scared to speak out. Colleagues used to point to the speaker in the staff-room, if a colleague was mouthing off about the regime. 'Watch your mouth, Gordon's listening,' they would say. Rowe used to enjoy showing his care workers the powers of his snooping devices. Often, he would confront them about complaints they had made behind closed doors, and enjoy their embarrassment at being found out.

It wasn't just technology that he used to spy on his staff and residents. Rowe designed the whole regime to prevent careless talk. He selected a small group of favoured and able residents—including John F and John M—to be his eyes and ears.

Their job was to tell him what the residents and staff were up to. They would tell Rowe if one of the care assistants had disobeyed his instructions and given a resident an extra cup of tea after lunch. One woman, who was in her fifties, was hauled up before Rowe because she had bought a packet of cigarettes during a shopping trip to Slough with one of 'Gordon's Girls', his small group of favoured female residents.

Malcolm*, who worked briefly at Stoke Place and Stoke Green, said: 'It was obvious that John F and John M had been brain-washed. John M wouldn't move unless Gordon had given him permission. He was Gordon's own little in-house surveillance camera. He had a walkie-talkie and everything. He would stand at the gate and take notes of the numbers of staff cars, when they came in and when they went out, and would tell Gordon Rowe what time they started and finished work.' He would even stand and watch the staff during lunch, and then tell Gordon how much they had eaten and how long they had taken.

'There was a lot of back-stabbing there, a hell of a lot,' Susannah told me. 'He told the clients to spy on the staff and on each other. None of the clients told you anything for about a couple of years, until they thought you were really trustworthy. There was gossip going around, but we didn't really know if it was real or not. Gordon was so clever... so convincing.'

Gary Moreton, another former care worker, who had discussed the cruelty of the regime with colleagues, agrees. 'Gordon was convincing and he convinced them that I was the trouble-maker. He could sit you down and talk to you for an hour and by the end of it you would think: "He's got a point."'

But it wasn't just the spying and the clever allocation of privileges and punishment that helped Rowe keep control. He also knew how to intimidate residents and staff by showing off his powerful friends. His best trick was to invite pals from Slough police for social visits, or arrange trips to Slough police station. Staff at Longcare believed there was no point filing a complaint about Rowe with Slough police.

It was important that Gordon's employees knew he had friends in high places. The more people who knew how important his friends were, the easier it was for him to force them into silence.

When Rowe's police mates came to visit, they would stand in reception, the best-decorated room in the mansion house. Pictures hung on the wall, the window frames were freshly painted and the carpet was less than ten years old. Gordon would make sure he was the centre of attention. He would tell his police friends a risqué joke or two, tell them how good he was to his residents, how he thought of them as his own family. Most importantly, he would make sure his staff knew exactly who his guests were.

Rowe knew his connections would raise other doubts in the minds of his staff. After all, if he had so many friends in the police, he couldn't be that bad a bloke, could he? Maybe he's right, they would think. Maybe this is the best way to treat these people. After all, he's been a social worker for 30 years. He must know what he's doing.

It was probably naivety on their part, rather than any deliberate attempt to help Rowe maintain his regime, which persuaded one or two officers to help him out with little favours. They didn't know they were merely a small part of a larger puzzle and that they, too, were being used.

19. Horse Potatoes

> 'Alan, who has a mental age of 18 months, could not tell anyone about his misery or the pain he was in... he was locked in an unheated attic room at the London Road residential care home, left curled up on a plastic-covered chair in a small, ripped T-shirt, lying in his own urine and faeces... Alan, dumped by his own county of Essex in the Northamptonshire home in 1989... had not received a single visit or inquiry from Essex since his care package was agreed... ten years ago.'
>
> *The Observer,* April 1, 2001

1999
DOROTHY: There was this boy and his name was Gary T and he was a very nice boy actually and he couldn't speak. And one day he was late for breakfast and he didn't have no breakfast so he had to go straight out in the garden and he was very, very hungry. So they used to keep horses and they gave the horse potatoes to the horses and Gary T pick one up and start eating it. So the gardener reported him to Gordon Rowe and at dinner time when everybody was sitting down to a lovely dinner, all Gary T had was this rotten potato on his plate. And Gordon Rowe said to him: 'Here, if you like eating potatoes so much, Gary T, then eat that one.' And so I took pity on him and I had this doggy bag under the table and I was just eating. When Gordon Rowe turned away... I would fill the bag full of stuff for Gary T. I took him aside and

said, 'here, Gary, take this, don't say nothing to Gordon Rowe.'

Then there was Jackie G. She would literally scream at the meal table because she was petrified of Gordon Rowe and his common law wife... so anyway, if she screamed they told her to keep quiet else they would put her down the bottom of the stairs and make her stand up to eat her food. So poor Jackie G would scream and she was pushed outside and made to stand outside in the cold and the rain to eat her food.

So one day I was very, very sick and I was drifting away into another world. I didn't even have enough energy to get out of bed to get out of my own vomit. So then this nice lady, Pat, came by. She said to me, 'shall I make your bed Dot and make you comfortable?' So I said, 'yes, please.' And she only got the top cover off when Angela Rowe came up and she told Pat to get out of the room that she would do it herself. She made me get up and make the bed and she made me make myself a cup of tea and then when I had it I was vomiting again and I lay there very sick indeed. So it came round to meal times and Gordon Rowe shouted up the stairs, 'get up, else you don't have nothing to eat at all.' So I didn't have the energy to get up and I still laid there. It was only after a few days that I had the energy to pull myself out of bed and get as far as top of the stairs and then I couldn't walk down the stairs and somebody came up to help me and Gordon Rowe said, 'get away from her, she can do it herself, she's only acting up.' So, anyway, I had to literally pull myself down on my hands and knees right down to the living-room and I didn't have the energy to hold a cup of tea. And so this nice staff, his name was Andrew and he was Irish, and he put the cup in my hand and cupped my finger round it and he held the cup for me and that's when I thought, well, not all people are not compassionate. But I was still full of the hate for Gordon Rowe.

1993

Longcare was run like a correctional facility, as if the residents were there to be punished. They were not free to come and go as they pleased, the food was poor and there wasn't enough of it, and physical punishment was a constant threat. They shouldn't expect too much, they learned, because they didn't deserve anything.

In Gordon's mind, the residents were the lowest of the low and should be grateful if they were fed and housed at all. He had been influenced very strongly by what he had learned in his years at Broadmoor. Rowe used to tell staff at Longcare how lucky the residents were to have him. 'Who else would look after them?' he would say.

On one occasion, according to a member of Longcare staff, *Michael S* had been sweeping up bird-droppings from the driveway and was sheltering under the trees from the rain with some of the other male residents. When Rowe saw this, he ordered them all back to work. Michael asked if he could go to one of the Longcare 'workshops' instead. As a punishment, Rowe dragged him by the collar to a patch of grass near his cottage and forced him to dig a hole in the ground.

When Michael knocked on the cottage door to say he had finished, Rowe came out to inspect the hole and decided it was not deep enough. He filled it in and ordered Michael to dig it again, giving him a parting slap on the back of his head. This, apparently, happened several times before Rowe was satisfied with the depth of the hole.

A movement caught Norman's* eye as he passed the window. A resident on the grass, arms and legs moving in jerks and jumps. An epileptic seizure.

He saw Lorraine's short, stocky figure march out towards the man. She walked up to him and stopped, looked down, but didn't bend. From the trees, Norman saw Gordon stride quickly across the lawn towards them.

Gordon stopped on the other side of the man and nestled his foot underneath his chest, then quickly flipped him over onto his side. He glanced across at Lorraine and said something. Lorraine nodded and she and Gordon turned and walked towards the house, leaving the man to finish his seizure on the grass.

These weren't isolated incidents. Most members of staff could point to several occasions when they had witnessed Rowe treat residents like this.

'The strange thing was that Gordon gave me the impression that he did care about the residents,' Steve* would tell me. 'I happened to mention to him one day that it must be a very profitable business. He turned round and said to me: "It's not a business to me. I like to look on it as a family home."'

Rowe could do this. Convince his staff that he cared about the residents, even while they watched him treat them like dirt. He was in command and he had the certificates and CV to back up his position.

Staff like Steve had heard rumours of serious abuse, but had witnessed maybe just a single kick up the backside, as well as instances of cruelty which Rowe would explain away as the kind of strict, disciplinarian regime which worked well at Broadmoor. Steve and others like him justified their inaction by telling themselves that they could either quit and abandon the residents they cared about, or stay on and make sure that at least one person was looking out for them. Money, of course, was another factor.

'At that time, with unemployment as it was, it was a difficult decision to just walk away,' Steve told me. 'And you had this feeling of protectiveness. When you walked in in the morning they would give you this feeling that they needed you. It was very difficult to just walk away from that. In the end, the reason I did walk away was that I was under so much pressure that I had to leave, and I went to sign on.'

1989

Gordon had bought Stoke Green House in 1987. It was on the other side of the main road from Stoke Place, about 50 yards from the entrance, and Gordon used it to house some of the more able residents. It was smaller and more relaxed than Stoke Place, and further away from Gordon. However, if any Stoke Green residents showed signs that they had become too friendly with the staff, they were immediately transferred back across the road.

Any residents who misbehaved were also transferred to Stoke Place, Gordon's punishment house. They would return a couple of weeks later, heavily drugged and hardly able to stand up straight. It happened to *Ben*. He had a habit of opening the washing machine late at night to get his clothes out, so he could have them by his bed in the morning when he woke up. But sometimes he opened the machine when it was still full of water. On one occasion, he flooded the laundry, and Lillian Lowe, the duty care assistant, called over to Stoke Place for help. Desmond Tully rushed over and he and Ben had a tussle on the stairs. Desmond dragged him over to Stoke Place.

When he came back a few weeks later, Ben had stopped running about all over the house and was hardly able to summon the energy to get out of a chair.

It happened all the time. When one of the residents became too boisterous, cheeky, or showed signs of refusing to bow to Gordon's authority, he would drug them up with Largactil or other drugs used to control psychosis. Of course, they weren't psychotic, but there wasn't much they could do about it.

Drugs such as Largactil can cause serious side-effects, such as difficulty talking or swallowing, muscle spasms of the head and neck, drooling, rashes, and uncontrollable movements of the body. But Gordon Rowe, with his experience of working at Broadmoor, easily convinced his staff, and other professionals, that these drugs were essential to treat the 'symptoms' displayed by his residents. He was the expert.

Debbie was another of the care workers who came forward later to describe what she had seen while working for Gordon Rowe. She, in fact, was one of those who tried anonymously to tip off the authorities.

'Debbie, get over here now. It's an emergency. Rebecca's* parents are here for a surprise visit, and…'

'Sorry, Desmond, I've got a house full of residents and there's just two of us on duty.' Debbie shook her head as she listened to Desmond rant.

'Get over here now and pretend you only popped over the road for a minute or two. They're in reception and I'm the only one here. Rebecca's been in her room for a fortnight, as a punishment for messing around with the boys. She'll need a wash.' He hung up.

Debbie shook her head, and grabbed her handbag and keys.

Something nagged her as she ran up the stairs to the first floor of Stoke Place, some little voice that warned her: 'This will not be good.' As she opened the door to Rebecca's room, the first thing she noticed was the smell: a rank, festering odour, sharp and pungent. Then she saw Rebecca's slight form in the far corner, her head hidden behind a blood-stained curtain.

There were faeces everywhere, on the curtains, the bed, smeared in a long trail across the carpet. But there was more. The staff had forgotten to give Rebecca her Pill. There was menstrual blood everywhere, most of it congealed on Rebecca's night-dress, which was crusted up with shit and dried blood and torn along one side. Her feet were bare and also covered in blood. She sat curled up, sobbing quietly, clutching the curtain she held over her face.

Debbie looked at the room, at Rebecca, and thought of her parents waiting downstairs. For one moment, she thought of showing them how their daughter was really being looked after. Instead, she walked slowly across the room. 'Let's get you cleaned up,' she said.

Later, when incidents like these became public knowledge, no-one could understand why the residents had not complained to their own families.

They seemed to see Gordon as a kind of second father. He punished them when they were 'naughty' and rewarded them when they were good. They accepted it, because they had learned from birth to rely on other people. Their survival at Longcare depended upon submission to the whims of Gordon Rowe. All of them were threatened or punished in some way; either by Gordon telling them they would be sent back to Botley's Park or 'sent away' if they were 'bad', or by beatings, or by threats of violence to loved ones. There were also rewards for 'good' behaviour: holidays, trips to clubs and to the seaside, and extra food.

'They all respected him,' says Susannah, another former care worker. 'They called him Daddy.' Most of the residents seemed to believe that they deserved the punishments inflicted on them. Michael had been locked in his room for days for some 'offence'. When Susannah slipped upstairs to check on him, he pleaded: 'I'll be good, I'll be good. Honest, I'll be good.'

Many of those who did try to alert their families to the abuse could not make themselves understood. Their reluctance to return to Stoke Place was seen as a wish to stay at home with their parents. They were said to be 'playing up'. Most of them were too scared to do anything but nod and grin when asked whether everything was all right at Longcare. Others, just as tragically, had no idea that what was being done to them was wrong.

20. A Walking Christmas Tree

> 'When you look at what the court has said referring to people with learning disabilities…what you see is nothing. There really have been no cases of any significance whatever before the European Court of Human Rights. Why have there been no cases when the level of abuse, the level of discrimination is awesome? We are in serious danger of perpetuating a system where the powerful have rights, but the vulnerable do not have rights, although on paper they are there.'
>
> Luke Clements, senior research fellow at Cardiff Law School; extract from a speech made to the Law and Justice for People with Learning Disabilities conference, organised by the Law Society and the Department of Health; March 30, 2001

1999
DOROTHY: *Gordon Rowe would also commit fraud with the residents' money. Well, I found out that because somebody used to*

send me cheques: £300 cheques, £400. But he always used to say: 'I will look after it. Shall I look after it, Dot, and put it in the bank to save you from standing up?' So he would play me against my cerebral palsy, but he didn't realise he couldn't play me against my brain. So he put it in the bank for me, but then I found out later it was a bank that Angela Rowe used. And then he used to say, 'I will put it in the bank for you and you can come and look at the books now and then and see how much interest you are getting.' So a couple of times I used to go in the office and say, 'Gordon Rowe, can I have a look at the books?' So he used to say, 'No, you can't, they are locked away somewhere. They are over in my cottage somewhere. I'll get them later on.' But then he used to forget to get them. So that's how I triggered on that there was something wrong with that.

Angela Rowe, she would dress up like a dog's dinner in mutton, like a flamin' mutton really. That's where the money was going. She had fur coats, she had pearls, she had diamonds, she was like a flippin' walking Christmas tree, only you put lights on her. Gordon Rowe hated me taking the mickey out of her like that.

She was going out and she came in with her fur coat on and dripping with diamonds and perfume an' that and she had all this make-up on, so I turned round to Jimmy and said, 'Put a couple of feathers up her arse and she would be a peacock.' Gordon Rowe didn't like that sort of thing. She was his common-law wife and that was it.

JP: Where did you get your clothes from?

DOROTHY: I couldn't afford new clothes. Everything was second-hand. I got them out of second-hand shops.

1989

In the first few years, there was always enough soap and toilet rolls to go round. But Gordon and Angela became greedy as they realised how much money they could make from the business. Maybe it had always been the plan to squeeze every last penny out of Longcare. Maybe Gordon just noticed how lax the council's inspection regime was. Whatever the explanation, as the years passed, food and toiletries were cut or rationed. But it wasn't just saving money; it was making money, too.

One night a week, the residents used to have fish and chips. They all paid for a full portion from their allowance, but only a favoured few received full servings. The rest received half a sausage and a few chips. A few always went without as a punishment. With nearly seventy residents at the two homes, this added up to a sizeable amount of 'chip money'. And then there were the videos. Gordon sometimes showed some of the residents a film as a treat. They were his tapes, from his own collection, but every Longcare resident was charged a few pounds for the 'rental'.

Angela was just as bad. She became furious at how many toiletries were being 'wasted' by the residents, so she introduced a system where each member of staff was given a carrier bag containing a tube of toothpaste, a roll of toilet paper and a bar of soap. Each bag was used by several residents—sometimes a whole corridor—and had to last a month. If the toilet paper ran out, Angela would ration extra supplies to two sheets a day. Soon, staff were finding faeces stains on the curtains. Some of the residents even resorted to using their face flannels to wipe themselves.

On one occasion, Angela ordered staff to collect all the bits of soap from the bathrooms and boil them up to make new bars. The 'new' bars fell apart almost immediately.

Staff often resorted to bringing in toiletries from home to make up for what Angela refused to provide.

Gordon Rowe's talent for making money from his residents was not only restricted to cost-cutting, rationing and chip money.

The more capable residents were used as part of Gordon's personal workforce. The women helped him and Angela with their cleaning, ironing and washing-up. The men were part of the 'working lads', the physically able male residents who were capable of working in the grounds. At first sight, the working lads sounded like a good idea. Give the men some exercise, let them do something useful, learn some skills. Better out in the fresh air than sitting around in an armchair watching television.

Rowe had talked about the 'working lads' in his letter to South Bucks councillors in 1983. It was all part of the supervised 'training' to be offered by Longcare. It sounded plausible enough, and so it seemed to many of the staff. Social and educational training, Rowe called it, disguising its true identity with a vaguely academic label. It was a tactic he frequently used to mislead the more naïve members of his staff. Describing a punishment as a 'behaviour modification technique', for instance.

But even if there was some vague educational or social benefit to a spot of gardening, it was twisted, as everything was twisted at Stoke Place. The men were expected to stay outside in poor weather, sometimes even when it was raining. It was more like a chain gang than occupational therapy. They learned nothing and wore unsuitable clothing. Many of the men could do little but clutch a hoe or a rake and stand outside, wearing a thin pair of trousers and an open-necked shirt, just about managing to move the tool backwards and forwards across the grass.

But for the most able men, there was real work to be done.

Rowe admitted to neighbours in a letter that he was bringing over 'a few of his more able lads' to help speed up the work on the extension to his large detached house in an exclusive Windsor cul-de-sac. He seemed to instinctively know that he would get away with it, and made little attempt to cover his tracks.

John F, who had a real talent for painting, and had worked as a decorator before he came to Stoke Place, decorated many of the bedrooms and hallways. He even used his own brushes and bought overalls with his own money. John also helped the builders and decorators who renovated Stoke Green House. Rowe didn't pay him for his help.

Bob spent a lot of his time at the Rowes' cottage in the grounds of Stoke Place. He cleaned, groomed the dogs, cooked their meals and looked after their son, Ben, who called him 'Butler'. Bob was often beaten by Angela and Gordon Rowe. Again, he wasn't paid for his work.

Rowe made use of Bob and the two Johns to help out his friends in the police force. John M told later how he had been taken to the home of a police officer to help with 'landscaping' work in his garden. He and the others had also been taken to the homes of the same officer and one of his colleagues, to help them decorate. They were paid a pittance for their work.

John M, another of the favoured working lads, worked on the extension. He was sexually assaulted by Gordon, who kicked him, threw chairs at him and pushed him down the stairs. Gordon warned him that he would have to leave Stoke Place if he told anyone what he was doing. Years later, John cried as he told his mum: 'I couldn't tell you, mum, because I thought it would upset you.'

There were other ways in which Rowe financially exploited his 'family'. Benefits payments disappeared into Rowe's bank account. Presents bought by relatives mysteriously vanished. Over the years, stereos, televisions and pieces of jewellery all disappeared. Whenever Rowe was questioned about their whereabouts, he would say they were 'broken' or 'in storage'. Clothes, too, went missing. New pairs of trainers, coats and jackets, designer jeans. Anything valuable always seemed to be misplaced.

The residents would return home for weekends dressed in borrowed, dirty and torn clothes. When quizzed, Rowe would always have an excuse.

Rowe already received hundreds of pounds a week in fees for each resident (£395 per week in 1989), and jacked up the profit margins by cutting back on staff, food and toiletries. He had probably worked out in Somerset how easy it would be to milk the system.

He made huge sums of money, enough to finance a holiday home in Florida, a boat, a Rolls Royce, a sports car, jewellery and fur coats for his wife, a Ferrari for his son, round-the-world cruises, homes for himself and his son in Windsor, as well as the mortgage-free purchase of Stoke Green House in 1987 and a number of other satellite homes in Slough.

Chris George says it took Rowe less than a year before he began to make serious money. 'We never thought we would get the House back, because Gordon was making so much money,' she says.

Even discounting the illegal siphoning of residents' funds and possessions, the Rowes were making a fortune. Longcare's official accounts show that, in 1984, the company made a profit of £37,845. The following year, this leapt to £103,864. At the time, the shares in the company were held by Gordon Rowe, Angela Adams and Raymond Beck, although Beck's 2,000 shares would soon be transferred to Nigel Rowe. These profits didn't include the salaries Gordon and Angela were drawing from Longcare Ltd.

By 1990, for instance, Gordon, as chairman, was being paid £72,053 a year, with the highest paid director (one of the Rowes, although it is not clear which one), earning £88,547. In 1991, Gordon was paid £85,095 as chairman, with the highest paid director earning no less than £104,696. These sums of money were far too high to be made from a normal care home. They were only the sums that went through the books. The money Rowe made on the side can only be guessed at.

There was nothing to stop Gordon Rowe defrauding the residents of Longcare. The county council's annual inspections never came close to revealing the fraud and theft, even though, in 1991, a council inspector told Longcare that too much of the residents' money was being kept in a company account. Gordon was also told that his wife should not be responsible for the personal savings accounts of residents who couldn't look after their own finances. At the time, she was the 'appointee' for nearly all such accounts. The following year's inspection discovered that he had not taken the slightest bit of notice and Angela was still the appointee for all but one of the residents.

There was never any danger that Gordon Rowe's scams would be uncovered. Any relatives' concerns were brushed aside, Slough police were on-side, the county council was incompetent and toothless, and the staff naïve and intimidated. Rowe could sit back and watch the money flood in.

21. The Railway Carriages

'Earlier this year a known paedophile walked free from a Crown Court after the second legal action against him in twelve months collapsed on the grounds that the victim was not considered a 'reliable witness'. In that instance the alleged victim, a young man, was eighteen years old at the time of the assault. So what was the problem? He suffers from severe learning difficulties and has the mental age of a 12-year-old child.'

The Times, November 14, 2000

1991
DOROTHY: *It was twelve o'clock on a Sunday and Jimmy had gone home for a little break. We were living in a little group home [by the front gate at Stoke Place]. I said something to one of the staff and threatened to let it all out what Gordon Rowe was doing to the residents. I didn't know he was going to go back and tell Gordon Rowe. And that's what he did.*
They picked us up for our dinner at one o'clock and then when I came back I sat down. I put a video on, I was putting some name-tapes on some socks of another resident and then it was two o'clock by then. Sylvia said to me, 'Is it two o'clock yet, Dot?' and I said, 'I think so. Go and put the kettle on and make two cups of tea.' So anyway, she was in the kitchen, she put the kettle on and we heard three great knocks on the door. Then I wouldn't answer the door because I had a vague idea who it was. So about a minute or so later the knocks came again: three great big ones. So Sylvia got frightened, she answered the door and in strode this Gordon Rowe, kicking the front door open and come into the living-room. So he says, 'Dorothy Abbot, I hear you've got something to say to me.' So I said, 'Yes, I hate you. I hate what you're

doing to the residents.' I saw these scissors so I picked them up and Gordon Rowe turned round and he caught my wrist and he made me drop the scissors. I said to him, 'I nearly killed you, Gordon Rowe'. And if I didn't have cerebral palsy, I would have stabbed him. But he pushed me down on the ground and he didn't even allow me to get up to walk. First of all he pulled me down a great doorstep on my back. So the front door smashed and he did get me down the step eventually and my fingers were rubbed to the bone. I had very long hair and he got hold of the little bits at the back of me hair, he pulled my head right back right across the gravel. And then I had this pink blouse on and it was changing colour from pink to red virtually because of the blood I was losing. And he pushed me down on the grass, which was wet, and I was shivering with shock, and hypothermia was also working in. So I broken off a pair of glasses and I thrown them at him and I said, 'There, Gordon Rowe, I'm not frightened of you.' So he tried to pull me and I ripped all the buttons on his shirt and these fingers were getting more and more rubbed down. I had blood clots in my hair and it was like the ordinary bloodbath out there.

1992

The residents were all treated differently. It was like a pyramid, with Gordon's favourites at the top, and people like David at the bottom. The favoured few were given treats and trips out, in return for doing favours and jobs for Gordon. Even though all of the residents paid for the outings, Gordon would tell his 'guests' he had paid for them himself. 'Gordon's taking us to a nightclub,' they would tell visitors. 'Gordon's taking us on a boat-ride.'

To the residents, Rowe was playing the part of the loving father. To his staff and outsiders, he was furthering the myth of the good-hearted, generous care home-owner who cared deeply about his 'family'. But those residents who didn't play the game were made to suffer. David was one such resident.

David had been brain damaged at birth and was only able to communicate through actions or grunts. This made him extremely vulnerable and a satisfying target to a bully like Rowe. David was also incontinent. Whenever Gordon heard about it, he would fly into a rage. David probably didn't know what was going on. He just had to stand there and take the punishment.

Gordon often slapped David when he 'messed himself'. Sometimes, he hit him so hard he knocked him down. He told the care workers that

David only messed himself to get attention, and there wasn't really anything wrong with him. You have to be strict, he said, or they take advantage. Staff told me how, on at least one occasion, Gordon hosed David down with cold water in the yard at Stoke Place after one of these episodes of incontinence.

Rowe knew he couldn't hit residents where a bruise would look suspicious. He knew the difference between 'accidental' and 'non-accidental' bruising from his days at Broadmoor, where beatings were an accepted practice. A bruise to the elbow or knee could be explained away as an accident, the kind of thing that happens to a clumsy disabled person from time to time. But bruises to the back or kidneys were a different matter and might arouse the suspicion of a social worker or relative. So he was careful.

About fifty or so yards from the end of the mansion was a wood. It started with a few scattered trees, but grew deeper and darker as you walked further in. Through the wood ran one of Rowe's little toys, a narrow gauge railway. Rowe loved to show it off when he held open days or threw charity functions to raise money for the residents (the money vanishing into Rowe's bank account). And on a rusty siding in a little clearing in the middle of the wood, sat a row of dark green railway carriages. It was towards these carriages that Gordon would drag David, returning alone. If he passed a care assistant in the corridor, he would say: 'Well, that's that sorted out. David has to have his dinner on the doorstep again. I've given him some of my psychology.'

The violence was part of the daily routine. It could be anything from a slap on the back of the head to a kick up the backside, a punch in the stomach to a severe beating in the wood. Gordon handed out his physical punishments like vitamin pills. He told staff they were an essential part of the discipline. Without the slaps and the kicks, he said, the whole place would descend into chaos. He told one care assistant, who had just watched him slap a resident across the back of his head for spilling his cereal: 'We have to show them who is boss. We have to show them who is in charge.'

For some of the residents, every day became a never-ending exercise in trying not to upset him. Cringing obedience, sucking-up, timid deference to Big Dada, these were the tactics adopted to avoid beatings. Often, even this wasn't enough.

Staff witnessed many of the less brutal physical attacks, but some of the more serious assaults were carried out in secret, in the woods, or in

Rowe's cottage in the grounds of Stoke Place. Rowe tied one resident to a tree and hosed him down, because of his incontinence. Another had been tied to the back of a tractor.

There were rumours among the staff about the fierceness of some of the beatings, but it was easier to turn away. They knew Rowe had threatened a colleague with legal action for making 'allegations' against him. They also knew he had many friends within Slough police. What was the point of risking their job when they didn't have any concrete evidence and weren't going to be believed anyway? And it wasn't as if the residents knew what was happening to them. No sense, no feeling.

Besides, Rowe was always able to justify his actions, often by referring to his training at Broadmoor, or pointing out his long career as a mental health nurse and social worker. He had the qualifications to prove it, and he could disguise the abuse in fancy words, convincing his staff that what he was doing was therapy, not abuse.

He also seemed somehow to instinctively know how far he could go in public, and when he needed to retire to a private place to dish out a beating.

He had already neutralised the threat of Slough police and he knew from long experience how easy it was to evade the limp hand of Buckinghamshire social services. Behind the high walls of Longcare, Gordon Rowe was king. And he knew it.

22. Gordon's Girls

> 'The abuse of vulnerable people in institutions and the community is a real problem and one that should not be underestimated. Our conference heard that many learning impaired people regard sexual abuse as a normal and expected part of life: a devastating concept.'
>
> Home Office consultation paper, *Setting the Boundaries: Reforming the Law on Sex Offences*, July 2000

1999
DOROTHY: One girl, her name was Sarah*, and she would come up to the classroom and she would start crying. And then that happened about

a week. I was getting her confidence in me and she would tell me and the result was that Gordon Rowe was having sex with her. And the teacher there was saying to her, 'stop crying, be quiet, don't be stupid, Gordon wouldn't do that'. But when it came out, Gordon was having sex with her. One day she was so hysterical, she said to me, 'Gordon Rowe has really hurt me,' and the next month she left. I don't know if he made her pregnant or what. She was gone to another place.

1990
Many of the female residents of Longcare were desperate for lives like those they saw around them, of their cousins, sisters, family friends, of women they saw on television. They wanted a boyfriend of their own, a husband, a home, a baby.

This was particularly true of the younger, more able female residents, the women nicknamed 'Gordon's Girls' by the staff. Residents like Janet Ward. Gordon had told her they were going to buy a house together. He said he was going to divorce Angela and marry her, because he loved her.

Rowe was able to see inside the heads of these female favourites. As he had said about the residents of The Old Rectory in a letter to South Bucks council in 1983: 'They all have their own individual personalities, their likes and dislikes, their fears, hopes and aspirations.' Rowe knew the 'fears, hopes and aspirations' of Gordon's Girls and used bribes, threats and violence to twist them out of shape and gratify his darkest urges.

Gordon believed he could do what he liked to his 'family' behind closed doors. If any of his victims complained to a relative or member of staff—despite the threats he had made—he would dismiss the claims as delusions, fantasies or grudges.

Many of the staff had tales to tell of how they had met female residents returning to their rooms hot, flustered and sweaty, hours after they should have been in bed. When pressed, they might admit they had been at the cottage with Gordon. This happened to Susannah, who had quizzed Susan, one of 'Gordon's Girls', when she disappeared during bath-time. When she returned, red-faced and out of breath, she eventually told Susannah that she had been with Gordon.

'She looked at me and said, 'He sup me,' and pointed between her legs. 'He sup me.' I put two and two together. After that, I never let her out of my sight, and she was always the last to be bathed. I tried to tell her to tell her mum. Then when her mum came, I said, 'Susan's got something to tell you,' but she didn't tell her. Part of me thought to try and get help. The other part of me said if I do that I will lose my job and she will never get any help. I thought, how could anyone believe me that there's something wrong? All of us were caught. People were always leaving Longcare, saying, 'I'm going to report them, I'm not having this.' I said: 'Please, do it.' But nothing happened. A cook, a cleaning lady, a few carers, they all said they would do it. That's why we have got such terrible guilt. It will never leave us.'

Lillian looked up and saw the clock showed 10.45pm. She walked through to the hall and saw Gordon Rowe stepping quietly up the stairs. She coughed loudly and he stopped, turned and smiled.

'Evening, Lillian.'

'Is anything wrong?' she asked.

He laughed. 'No, I have to speak to two of the girls. They were raising hell in the classroom, so I thought I'd better come over and speak to them. They'll be good once I've sorted them out.'

He turned without saying another word and trotted up the stairs, humming. She heard a door open above and the sound of his voice. The door closed and the house was silent again.

She didn't know how long she sat there. Eventually, she pushed back the chair and walked through to the hall. She heard nothing but the faint sound of Gordon's voice, muffled and fuzzy. She took a couple of steps up the stairs and stopped again, listening. Again, all she could make out was the sound of his voice, but too dull and indistinct to hear the words.

She saw the handle turning and the door slowly open. Gordon stumbled out of the room, but didn't see her. He was looking down, concentrating on zipping up his trousers, his hair stuck to his forehead with sweat, his face red and puffy. When he looked up, he saw Lillian standing a few feet in front of him.

'Right, that's it. She'll be good now,' he said, laughed once, and brushed past Lillian down the stairs.

A couple of weeks later, Lillian was sat again in Stoke Green. She had just been upstairs to talk to two of the men, who had been having an argument about a book. After that, she had walked round the corridors to listen for any residents who might be out of bed.

She heard a loud creak coming from the stairs. She looked up from her magazine and saw Tracey, looking towards her, kneading her fingers and shaking her head from side to side.

Lillian got up and walked through to the hall.

'*Hello Tracey, can't you get to sleep?*'

Tracey's hair was matted and tangled, as though she had been pulling and playing with it. As Lillian drew closer, she also saw her fringe was damp and her eyes red and bleary.

'*What's the matter? Have you been crying?*'

The young woman didn't answer, just continued to shake her head and knead her fingers.

'*Come and sit down and tell me about it,*' *said Lillian,* '*If there is something bothering you, you must tell me. It will all be better once you've told someone what the problem is.*'

Tracey looked up at Lillian for the first time, and sobbed: '*I hate that Gordon.*'

Lillian felt her mouth dry up. '*Gordon? Why?*'

'*Does things. Don't like it.*'

'*What kind of things, Tracey?*'

Tracey shook her head, covered her face with her arms and rested them on the table in front of her, and said: '*Scared.*'

'*What? What are you scared about?*'

'*Have baby.*'

It was surprising how careless Rowe became around this time. Maybe he simply became over-confident. He had got away with it at The Old Rectory in Somerset.

He knew very well that it was almost impossible to secure convictions in such cases—most of his victims would not be able to give evidence in court, and the others would be torn to shreds in the witness box. Plus, he had his friends in Slough police. He still remembered how easy it had been to shake off the allegations in Somerset. He was confident he would never be caught. And if he was ever arrested, he was even more confident that he would never be convicted.

Many people with learning difficulties who have been raped or sexually assaulted find it impossible to come to terms with what has been done to them. Some attempt to cope by abusing drugs or alcohol, by developing eating disorders or harming themselves.

Burke and Bedard[1] concluded: 'The self-mutilation...may be the only way a person can communicate what the abuse was, and to suggest the emotional distress it is causing.' They added: 'Often, abused individuals are told by the abuser that their actions are the way people show that they 'love' one another—when such sexual interaction ends, the client may resort to self-harm in an attempt to gain someone's love and attention.'

It wasn't only Janet. So many of the women—and men—were raped or sexually assaulted by Rowe. Mostly he picked on his favourites among 'Gordon's Girls' and the 'Working Lads'. He attacked them in their bedrooms or in his cottage in the grounds of Stoke Place during the afternoons, when Angela was out shopping. They were given special privileges in return, such as visits to a nightclub or trips in his boat. If they objected, he used violence. John M would often be called over to the cottage during the afternoons. If he resisted the assaults, Rowe would throw chairs, punch and threaten him.

1992

Parvinder's face was often swollen with bruises. She always explained to staff that she had had a seizure and had fallen. 'Her face would be black and blue, but the rest of her body wasn't touched,' remembers Susannah, one of the care assistants. 'It looked as though she had been in a fight. I never saw her have a fit, but if I went off duty and came back, her face would be black and blue.'

It was late on a Saturday afternoon. Susannah was looking for Gordon. She left the reception area and walked towards the stairs, listening for his voice.

She heard her stumble before she saw her. As Susannah looked up, Parvinder fell into her arms, breathing hard, clinging to her for support. She propped her up, held her at arm's length and looked into her eyes. They didn't return her gaze, but stared through her, vacant, just allowing the arms to hold her up.

'Parvinder, what's wrong?'

There was no reaction. She continued to look through and past her.

'Parvinder?'

'OK,' she said, and shook her head. She leaned against the wall for support and pushed herself away and past, towards reception.

Susannah heard more steps. They were firmer, more confident, but were coming from the same direction. The stocky form of Gordon Rowe appeared around the corner. His face was flushed and he appeared out of breath, his white hair damp and sticky. He stopped as he saw Susannah.

'Gordon, there's a call for you.'

'Never mind that. Did you see Parvinder?'

'Yes.'

'Oh, good.' He hesitated. 'How did you find her?'

'She looked a bit dazed and upset,' said Susannah. 'What's wrong with her?'

'Nothing,' he said. 'Nothing medical.'

For Rowe, the humiliation of the people in his charge had to be even deeper.

He would often make 'Gordon's Girls' watch pornographic videos. They would all have to take their clothes off, and weren't allowed to leave the locked room until he gave them permission to go.

Then there were his 'films', in which he forced female residents to have sex with male residents while he filmed them. Afterwards, he would force the women to watch themselves 'perform' on the videos.

One of the men once told a member of staff: 'That Gordon Rowe's in trouble. I would like to burn his house down in Windsor. He's doing things to me. I will tell you one day.'

'Paul used to cry and get all upset,' another care worker told me. 'He used to say that if he had done anything wrong, he would have to do things… and Gordon would be stood there with his camera. John F used to say the same thing: that he had to do certain things… so that Gordon could use his camera. I believe they were genuine and scared, and just wanted somebody to talk to.'

It took so much courage for a resident to tell something like that to a member of staff, because they never knew whom they could trust. And the staff turnover was so high that by the time a resident got to like and trust a care worker, they had usually left for another job.

It wasn't as if Rowe pretended to be a saint. He was always talking about sex to the staff, and often told them how over-sexed the residents were. The inappropriate behaviour that resulted from the abuse he had inflicted was used to provide his own cover stories. He said this behaviour was a symptom of the resident's disability. He knew very well what nonsense this was, but most of the care assistants were so inexperienced that they didn't know any better.

As for the residents, it was probably in part the feeling of worthlessness that secured their silence. They believed that they had brought the attacks upon themselves by something they had done to provoke him. They deserved what Rowe was doing to them, because they had been told they were inferior to 'normal people'. Besides, there was so much confusion. Why was it happening? What was it, anyway? And, because Gordon was doing it, did that mean it was OK? Fear, pain, confusion, guilt, anger, all messed up by their inability to express their feelings about what was happening—even if there had been someone listening.

Sobsey and Doe[2] found in one study that many victims of sexual abuse felt it was 'useless' to report what was happening because they feared 'retribution' or being sent away from their home. The authors added: 'The experiences of those among this sample and elsewhere who reported the abuse to authorities and elsewhere suggest that such fears are often justified.'

But even this wasn't the end of the sexual perversions Rowe inflicted on the residents. Many of the Longcare staff couldn't bring themselves to believe that Gordon was actually raping the people he was meant to be caring for. Susannah heard rumours that he was forcing them to have sex with animals. 'I hoped it wasn't true,' she told me, 'because it made me feel sick.'

Another care assistant, Frances*, remembers: 'I saw an ad in the paper for carers. I had never done the job before. The first weekend I was there, I heard the most terrible rumours about him [Gordon Rowe], that he videos clients with animals having sex. The first thing I said was that these people must really hate him to say these things about him.' Lillian also remembered being told about forced bestiality by a resident.

None of the staff had ever seen Gordon Rowe having sex with a resident. He did it behind locked doors. How could they know for sure that that was what he was doing, and that the residents were not just making it up, or were confused about what had happened? So they gossiped, or tried to blank it out, or kept an eye on 'Gordon's Girls' when they worked a night shift. They couldn't risk their livelihood by making a complaint. They had bills to pay and children to feed. And maybe Gordon was just over-friendly. They couldn't be sure.

And so Rowe was free to continue as before, until, finally, a few members of Rowe's staff decided enough was enough.

1993

Rosie perched on the edge of her bed and stuck out her feet, pointing her toes. It was her favourite part of bath night, having Clare rub the cocoa butter cream in. Afterwards, Clare would draw up her chair and put her own feet on the bed, as Rosie returned the favour.

Tonight, though, was different.

Clare put her feet up, as usual. But rather than reaching for the tube of cream, Rosie sat there, on the edge of the bed, her hands kneading each other as though she was rubbing the cream in, even though her palms were empty. She didn't look at Clare, but down at the carpet.

'I got secret with Big Dada.'

Clare's feet thudded into the carpet. She remembered what she had seen after bathing another female resident. There had been bruising around the woman's anus, and she had been determined not to let it go, as most of her colleagues had told her to do. Instead, she had told Gordon that the bruises meant the woman had almost certainly been anally raped.

He blamed it on a cracked toilet seat. She remembered his words: 'The problem with you, my girl, is that you have done this new-fangled course and you want to find something wrong here. But if you did, you would be a very silly girl and you would never work in the care sector again.' The message couldn't have been clearer.

She had lately become ever more convinced that Gordon was responsible for the bruising, as he had been responsible for the incident in the classroom she had caught on her video camera, which had then been wiped by Gordon during the editing process.

By now a trickle of complaints had started to reach Bucks County Council.

It started with two anonymous telephone calls from a former member of staff in December, 1992. She had seen Gordon Rowe kick residents, punish them by making them eat outside, and order them to have cold showers. She had also heard that Rowe had sexually assaulted female residents.

A second former member of staff made similar allegations of neglect and ill-treatment two months later, followed by a third call a few days later. The following month, another former Longcare employee, Allan*, wrote a letter to Berkshire County Council, which was forwarded to Buckinghamshire. Allan, who had previous care experience, made further allegations of physical abuse and ill-treatment.

It was incidents like her conversation with Rosie that had persuaded Clare that she had to do something. She had already started to keep a diary of incidents, on the advice of Gary Moreton, who had already left Longcare. 'I had wanted to complain,' she said later, 'but I was seventeen and there was such a large staff there and no-one wanted to know. They would say: 'You can't say anything. We will lose our jobs. It's all right for you, Clare, but we have mortgages, we have got kids to feed.'

'It was a big step, and I was frightened of him [Gordon]. In the end, I spoke to Allan* and Gary. It was obvious that it was still going on. Then *Alison* had gone over to Gordon's cottage and came back with her top inside out and her bra done up wrong, and I thought, 'Oh, no.' And Rosie told me how he had stuck her deodorant inside her. I just thought it was wrong. My mum said, whatever I decided to do, she would stand by me.'

In July, 1993, the Buckinghamshire inspection unit heard that Clare wanted to join those members of Longcare staff who had talked to them about Gordon Rowe's regime. They called her and she agreed to meet them at home in Slough. 'It was very hush-hush,' she said. 'Then the police came and took me to Windsor police station under a different name. They had to take me there, because of the contacts Gordon Rowe had at Slough police station.

'Social services met me at home every week. I was seeing them in the morning and then going in to work at Longcare. It was making me quite ill.'

She gave a council inspector's card to a friend who also worked at Longcare. He called the inspection unit, and made a statement.

There are two questions worth asking in relation to the sexual abuse. Why did Rowe do it? And why was he not found out earlier?

There are no easy answers to the first question, only guesses. It is probable that, to do what he did, Rowe must have aroused by the unfettered power he held over the residents of Longcare, possibly even by their emotional immaturity and naivety. But it is plain above all else that to do what he did, he must have felt that their lives, their wishes, were worthless.

---

[1] Burke, Lillian; Bedard, Cheryl: Self-injury Considered in Association with Sexual Victimization in Individuals with a Developmental Handicap; The Canadian Journal of Human Sexuality, Vol 3(3), Autumn 1994.

[2] Sobsey, Dick and Doe, Tanis: Patterns Of Sexual Abuse and Assault; Sexuality and Disability, Vol 9, No 3, 1991.

INVESTIGATIONS

23. Serious Implications

> 'Big Brother, the television show which split the nation, was regarded by millions of viewers as bright, innovative, and exciting. Many more thought it was tacky, mundane and boring. But the cavortings of a bunch of extrovert nobodies locked in a custom-built house certainly appeared worthwhile yesterday when winner Craig Phillips—one of the programme's biggest show-offs—got serious. The bodybuilding bricklayer pledged his £70,000 prize from the Channel 4 show to a Down's Syndrome teenager who needs a heart and lung transplant in America. Joanne Harris has been refused treatment in Britain, prompting accusations that Down's children were being discriminated against.'
>
> *Sunday Express*, September 17, 2000

SIR/MADAM,
FOR OBVIOUS REASONS I AM UNABLE TO SIGN THIS NOTE. HOWEVER, I THINK IT IS AN ISSUE OF SOME IMPORTANCE. THERE APPEAR TO BE SERIOUS IMPLICATIONS, A POSSIBLE COVER-UP, AND NO SIGN THAT OTHER LOCAL GOVERNMENT OFFICES HAVE BEEN NOTIFIED ABOUT THIS MATTER. IT WOULD CERTAINLY WARRANT SOME FURTHER RESEARCH.
SINCERELY,
'CONCERNED'

Janice Raycroft had joined the *Slough Observer* nearly twenty years before as a young reporter. She was fiercely loyal to the paper, despite the steadily-increasing sense of doom surrounding its finances (it was sold a couple of years later to a Scottish newspaper group) and nothing stirred her blood more than fighting to stand up a good story.

The first move was to confirm with the council that the report was genuine. The second was even more obvious: get out to Longcare for a reaction.

The two Longcare homes nestled in Green Belt just a few hundred yards from the northern tip of Slough, and at the southern end of the leafy expanse of Buckinghamshire. In fact, Stoke Place Mansion House was just about the last building in Buckinghamshire before you reach the outskirts of Slough.

No-one at Longcare would comment on the leaked report. I was not the first reporter there, because we had been slow off the mark, and I received a frosty reception. There was no-one available to talk to me, according to the woman who answered the door.

My first impression was of a cold, ill-maintained, forbidding building. I had gained a brief glimpse inside the entrance hall, but had not seen a single resident.

I had driven past the high brick walls surrounding Stoke Place on many occasions over the previous nine months, but couldn't remember ever having noticed the entrance on the main road, Stoke Green, or even Stoke Green House, planted just a few feet back from the road.

I returned to the office to track down Gordon Rowe's home address. All we knew from the report was that he lived in Windsor. There were several G Rowes in the telephone book. The first lived in a small flat in Old Windsor, a village on the edge of Windsor Great Park. 'Rusty', though, couldn't talk to me about his brother, Gordon: he had Alzheimer's. His wife told me they didn't see much of Gordon. 'We don't even know where he lives,' she said.

The next addresses were in an exclusive, moneyed cul-de-sac on the western edge of Windsor: Harrington Close. There were two Rowes who lived on the right-hand side of the road, one at number ten, the other at twelve. I tried ten first. A woman answered the door. She knew nothing about a Gordon Rowe. She had never heard of him. She later turned out to have been the wife of Nigel Rowe, Gordon's eldest son. I tried next door, number twelve. This time, the door didn't even open. But when I returned to the office and telephoned the house, Gordon answered.

'I'm sorry, I've got nothing to say to you at all,' he said, and hung up.

Raycroft had by this time taken the report home to read thoroughly. She had also shown it to the *Observer*'s owner, Peter Lawrance. 'I was sickened,' she says. 'I wanted to go round and hit the people who had been doing these things. If I could have had them in front of me I would have given them a good kicking, and I think in his own genteel way that is how the proprietor felt.' She told Lawrance the report had 'serious implications' and could prove to be one of the *Observer*'s biggest stories.

'It made you angry: one, because it had happened; and two, because it was all in a secret report that was saying, 'how can we make this go away?' If it had happened to me, nobody would have been writing a secret report. I was just outraged.'

It was clear we were not going to get enough of a response from Longcare or Gordon Rowe to put us legally in the clear. But Raycroft was desperate to run the story, even though all three of our weekly rivals—who had also received copies of the report—did not publish stories that week.

This presented us with certain legal problems: the first was whether it was safe to print extracts from a confidential county council report we had no right to possess. The second and more serious was the risk of being sued for libel by Gordon Rowe. The report was not a public document and we had already received two faxes from Rowe's legal advisers, warning us that he *would* sue if we published stories based on the report.

'It was quite clear from the report that there were loads and loads of apparent witnesses, but all of them were terrified and anonymous to us,' says Raycroft. She knew she would need some serious legal advice. She called the paper's London solicitors, Mishcon de Reya.

Time was running out. If their libel lawyer advised us to shelve the story, we would have to follow his advice, no matter how much we wanted to run with it. A series of phone calls and faxes were exchanged between the *Slough Observer* and Mishcon's London office. Eventually, as Thursday's deadline approached, the libel lawyer called the editor.

The advice was simple: you can run the story, but you had better hope you get some witnesses to back up your allegations. 'If we published we had to go all out and then hope the witnesses came forward,' said Raycroft.

'I knew that if we didn't stand it up it would pull the *Observer* down and sink it. It's the only time in my career that I have taken that dangerous gamble, but it was worth it 100 per cent in the end.'

REIGN OF TERROR IS UNCOVERED

Secret report reveals a catalogue of torment and humiliation— handicapped people were kicked, punched and abused

MENTALLY handicapped adults were subjected to a horrific reign of terror at two residential homes, a top secret inquiry has concluded.

Today the Observer tells how a lengthy Bucks County Council investigation uncovered dozens of allegations that some residents of Stoke Place Mansion House and nearby Stoke Green House had been sexually assaulted, beaten and tormented between 1991 and last year.

At the centre of the investigation was Gordon Rowe, of Harrington Close, Windsor, former director and managing director of Longcare Ltd, the company that runs the homes, on the Slough and Stoke Poges border...

Slough and Langley Observer, Friday, September 16

On Friday morning, September 16, just a couple of hours after the paper was in the news stalls—*The Independent* had also run the story on its front page—the telephone rang in the newsroom. It was an ex-member of Longcare staff. He had read the story and he wanted to talk.

My initial reaction had been one of revulsion. But in those early days, this was aimed squarely in the direction of the 'perpetrators': Gordon Rowe, his wife Angela and Longcare manager Lorraine Field, who lived near the homes in Stoke Poges. It was only in the following weeks and months that the true scale of the abuse at Longcare began to fall into place.

For such an apparently shocking story, though, the reaction from our readers in Slough, South Buckinghamshire and Windsor was muted. There was no outrage. We were not swamped with letters calling for 'something to be done'. In fact, in the three-and-a-half years that I covered the story for the paper, we received only a handful of letters about the case. Most of these were from people with a vested interest in the story: politicians, voluntary organisations, relatives of Longcare residents. It took me nearly six years to understand why.

24. The Care Staff

> 'The TOPSS plan suggests some 83,000 people work in learning disability services, with around 75 per cent having no qualifications at all and many, especially managers, not having very relevant qualifications.'
>
> Extract from speech by James Churchill, Chief Executive of the Association for Residential Care, at a Training Organisation for the Personal Social Services conference, February 2, 2000

Interviewing former Longcare staff members about their time at the homes, the obvious question would always be: why didn't you tell the authorities? By the time the inspection unit finally launched its investigation, late in 1993, Rowe had been abusing residents for nearly 10 years.

It was easy enough to blame these care workers. But was that fair?

I talked in depth to fourteen former members of Longcare staff. Every one of them spoke about the atmosphere of threats and intimidation created by Gordon Rowe.

One ex-care assistant described Rowe as 'the sort of man whose presence made you feel afraid. There was a certain aura about him. I was very surprised that the clients looked up to him as a father figure, because he was very, very strict in everything he did. They would be so afraid when he walked into a room. 'Hello, Gordon. You want a cup of tea, Gordon?' they would say. They were all out to score points, to get in his good books, because they had to survive in that place.'

That sense of fear and menace was used to control staff as well as residents. One former employee said: 'He used intimidation to keep them quiet. I know for a fact that one or two staff who tried to complain got threatening phone calls. He was a very powerful man and he had some very powerful friends.' He talked openly about his 'contacts' and had made sure everyone knew he was a Freemason. His staff believed he had contacts at Bucks County Council and within the Conservative Party, of which he was briefly a member.

Care assistant Lillian Lowe was one of those who did not manage to lodge a complaint. When I asked her whether she regrets this, she told me: 'Yes, I do, but the staff had the impression that, because Gordon Rowe knew so many people in high places, they would not believe the likes of us and he would get away with it.'

Yet several care workers did report what they had seen to the authorities. Gary Moreton told me that a couple of staff went to Slough police station to lodge a complaint in the early 90s and were 'laughed out of the door'. They were told: 'Unless you have got any evidence, there is nothing we can do about it.'

This must have underlined the pointlessness of complaining. The staff knew about Gordon Rowe's connections. They were also scared of their boss and of what he might do to their careers.

But it wasn't just Gordon Rowe the care workers had to contend with. Rowe had cleverly created an atmosphere where back-biting and bitchiness among the staff were rife. One ex-care assistant told me: 'People hated each other. You could never rely on anyone, because what you said to one person would go straight back to Gordon. It got to a point where you didn't have any friends you could rely on.' Staff spied on staff, residents spied on staff and each other, and Gordon spied on everyone. The homes were festering pots of lies, deceit and paranoia.

If one of the staff looked as though he might cause problems, Rowe spread a little gossip, hinted at a bit of wrong-doing, or perhaps told other care workers their colleague was 'mad' or held a grudge. If that failed, he might try some subtle blackmail or explain that a resident's inappropriate behaviour was because he was 'over-sexed'.

One male care assistant, who worked for Longcare for seven months in the early 90s, told police that two senior Longcare managers, Ray Cradock and Nigel Rowe, had quizzed him about complaints he had made to other members of staff.

Gary Moreton worked at Stoke Place and Stoke Green for about two years, and finally left in March, 1992. He paints a vivid picture of the tricks Rowe used. 'He was very clever—he manipulated people in such a way that they would be unable to stand up against him. He got a kick out of playing mind games with the staff. Another thing he did was to offer staff money if they were in financial trouble. He knew they would never be able to pay him back.'

'He only ever employed people who desperately needed a job and had no experience of care work. He convinced them that his way was the way it was done—he openly told people that Longcare was run like a prison.'

Like Broadmoor, in fact. Rowe often told inexperienced care assistants that the violent 'techniques' they saw him use were accepted practice within the care industry.

The things Gary witnessed at Stoke Place slowly began to take over his personal life. Catriona, his wife, who also briefly worked at Longcare, remembers: 'He would come home and want to unwind, but we would end up talking about Gordon Rowe for hours, working out strategies to protect the residents. It was ridiculous.'

The mind games Gordon Rowe played on the staff were nothing to the ones he played on the residents. Gary Moreton says Rowe deliberately set out to humiliate them and break down their personalities until all signs of rebellion had vanished. Many felt so worthless they began to mutilate themselves with knives or razor blades. Then they were punished for that. If a member of staff complained, Rowe would take great pleasure in repeating the punishment time and time again, as if to say: 'That's what happens to the ones you try and stick up for.'

He told Gary Moreton how to whip their legs with wet towels. The advantage of this form of punishment—apart from the pain—was that it left no lasting marks. He told Gary on one such occasion: 'That will make them realise I mean business.'

It was this systematic humiliation of the residents that helped to create an atmosphere in which the daily abuses they were subjected to could pass without action or comment. Inexperienced care workers saw the way Rowe treated his clients and, even if only subconsciously, allowed it to reinforce their negative preconceptions about learning disabled people.

After about a year working at Longcare, Gary Moreton began a social work course and slowly learned the correct way to treat learning disabled people. It was at about this time, he says, that Rowe began to 'get sloppy'. Displays of violence against residents became more common and began to occur in the presence of more than one member of staff. Care workers who had dismissed the rumours began to believe that these things really were happening.

Gary took advice from his college tutors. They told him to be careful, to stand up to Gordon Rowe and complain when he saw something he didn't like. He thought about leaving, but decided it would be better to stay and try to protect the residents.

Eventually, Rowe called Gary to his office, produced six pages of 'allegations' Gary had made about him to other members of staff, and threatened to sue for defamation.

When Gary refused to retract the allegations, Rowe's façade of control and power started to crumble. He turned bright red and began trembling and sweating, avoiding the other man's eyes while he shuffled his papers. Gary offered to resign. That was the last thing Rowe wanted. He preferred his opponents to stay with Longcare, where he could keep an eye on them. Instead, Gary was transferred from Stoke Place Mansion House to Stoke Green.

Of course, not every employee disliked and feared Gordon Rowe. Many remained loyal. People like Lorraine Field, a former hospital cleaner, who had been promoted far above her abilities to care manager. Rowe also employed several members of his family, including Angela, Nigel, his brother Ted, one of his sisters and her husband.

Rowe often made sure he could trust those in senior positions by taking unqualified staff and training them himself, as he had with Desmond Tully and Lorraine Field. 'That's why Lorraine lasted so long,' said one ex-member of staff. 'She was seen as a "yes woman". If Gordon had told her to jump in the lake, she would have done it. If you asked her why, she would have said: "Because Gordon told me to."'

Tully was later to tell a court hearing that he was 'not proud of having worked there', and added: 'I carried out things I wasn't happy about. I was constantly employed to cover up situations. But we were limited in what we could do. It was Gordon's place, wasn't it?' Tully, who worked at Longcare for several months from 1983, and again for three years from 1987, added: 'You might say, "Why did you work there?" You have to know how to get out of there. It was not the easiest place to get out of.'

But scores of staff did leave Longcare. It took months before a resident would feel comfortable enough to confide in a care worker, and by that time they would probably have left for another job. Most of the trained care workers walked out of their jobs at Longcare almost immediately, once they realised what it was like, and there was also a high turnover among less qualified staff. It was a standing joke that, at one time or another, everyone in Slough had worked there.

Debbie, who worked as a care supervisor, lasted less than a year before quitting her job to go on the dole. 'It was making me ill. I had to leave, or I would have ended up doing myself in,' she told me. 'But I quit while Gordon and Angela were on holiday, because I didn't have the courage to do it while they were there. He would have talked me into staying.'

'The atmosphere was like walking into a factory,' said Monica. 'You couldn't wait to get out. I just feel sorry that I didn't do anything, that we weren't strong enough. But I think all of us were worried about what would happen to us.'

Rowe often told his employees how easy it would be to replace them. And he knew they would need a reference for another job. One young classroom assistant told me: 'We knew there were a lot of people out of work, so we had to toe the line. The way we dealt with it was to just close the classroom door and forget there was an existence outside the room.' Another young woman told me: 'It was like going into a factory. Input and output. Profit-making. We clocked in. We clocked out. As soon as five o'clock came, we were rushing to get out.'

Monica*, who worked for Longcare for five years from the late 80s, was another of the youngsters taken on by Rowe on YTS schemes. 'I am sure people say: "Why did you stay for five years?" But my parents put a lot of pressure on me, saying I couldn't leave unless I had another job to go to,' she told me.

She was young and inexperienced. For example, Rowe told her that David's incontinence was just 'attention-seeking' and he was to be put out in the garden as a punishment. How was she to know that this wasn't the way things were supposed to be done?

But there were incidents that were even more obviously wrong. She once saw Rowe tie David to a tree and leave him there because he 'messed himself'. Sometimes, she says, residents would scream in terror as they watched through a window as Gordon punished one of their friends. 'Gordon had such power, and not just over the residents, over the whole staff. I think some of us were frightened we would never get another job in the caring profession.'

Another trick Rowe used was to attack the credibility of the residents' parents, so his staff would not be tempted to confide in them. He even spread vicious lies about some of the families to his care workers, falsely accusing them of cruelty and abuse and inventing bizarre case histories for many of the residents to help cover his own tracks.

It was only the particularly strong-willed members of staff—and often those who were also taking outside social care courses—who could see through this fog of abusive, controlling behaviour. Fortunately, a small number of staff—including Clare Johnson—*did* find the courage to register a proper complaint, to make sure something was done. It was from this small group that the complaints that would eventually bring down Gordon Rowe were to come.

There had been a widespread certainty among Longcare staff for so long that no-one would be able to force the police or council to investigate Gordon Rowe. They assumed justice would never be done, so when, one Sunday evening in November 1993, one of the care assistants blurted out in a staff meeting that Buckinghamshire council had launched an investigation, the news was met with a stunned silence. It was broken by Longcare manager Ray Cradock. 'Investigating us? For what?' he asked.

Even before the inspection unit's probe had started, Gordon and Angela Rowe suspended themselves from Longcare. But Rowe employed a solicitor to interview each member of his staff and warn them of their obligation to maintain the company's confidentiality.

Three days before Christmas, the inspection unit was told that Gordon would retire at the end of the year. The following month, Nigel told staff in a memo how his father's retirement had been 'carefully planned' over the previous eighteen months. Angela would eventually resign as a Longcare director and employee on July 4, 1994.

Clare remembers the immediate effect of the inspection unit investigation. 'All of a sudden, everyone had pictures on their walls, everyone had a choice of food.' Despite this, Rowe's appointees were still in positions of power. Clare remembers Lorraine Field saying to her: 'Do you really think it's going to change?' and warning her: 'Don't you think your life is going to be a bit difficult here now?' 'I don't care,' Clare replied. 'I have achieved what I wanted to achieve.'

Clare left Longcare in February, 1994, in the middle of the inspection unit probe. She and others who had talked to the inspectors before the investigation was launched, paid for their bravery by receiving anonymous, threatening telephone calls from Gordon Rowe's henchmen. It was proof, perhaps, that those care workers who had been too scared to complain had had some justification for their concerns.

As the investigation dragged on well into the New Year, morale continued to plunge. Nigel Rowe threatened to sack any staff who gave confidential information to outsiders. They took that to mean the inspection unit. Nigel was rattled. So was Cradock, who told care workers in another memo that their standards were slipping.

The report was finally completed in June, 1994. Despite severe shortcomings in the investigation, the inspectors had gathered an abundance of evidence. The tone of the report was one of horror. Jennifer Waldron, head of the inspection unit, concluded that Gordon Rowe had been responsible for behaviour of almost unimaginable cruelty.

Nigel Rowe and Ray Cradock were predictably scathing about the report. They called it 'blatantly inaccurate' and said nearly every allegation had been made by staff with grudges against Longcare. They accused witnesses of collusion and cast doubt on their credibility. They said they believed the county council was conducting a 'witch-hunt' against Longcare and denied nearly every example of abuse detailed by Waldron's team. Nigel Rowe had been working with his father for years, ever since—with a short break in the mid-80s—he joined him as a care assistant in Somerset at The Old Rectory. Ray Cradock had been at the homes since 1990, when he began working for Longcare as a consultant.

Some of the care assistants admitted respect for Cradock. He boasted an impressive CV, with a social work career spanning 28 years, including spells in residential homes in Honduras and Guatemala and experience of conducting inquiries into abuse at other residential homes in Britain. He was also married to Gordon Rowe's first wife, Pat. He was originally employed as a consultant to Longcare in 1990, before his appointment as director of services in September, 1992, and, later, registered manager of the two homes.

Inevitably, the investigation hit the company hard, with the withdrawal of many of its clients over the next eighteen months. Eventually, two years after the inspection unit's report was leaked, Stoke Green House was closed, and the management of Stoke Place was passed to REACH, a new company unconnected with Longcare.

In a letter to relatives of residents in April 1996, Cradock spoke of the 'unsubstantiated allegations of abuse by former employees' and the 'life threatening letters and phone calls, intimidating police, social services and media activity, negative newspaper articles and television programmes' he and the company had been subjected to. He said Longcare had lost 70 per cent of its business. 'There is no doubt in our minds,' he said, 'that the authorities have closed ranks and made it impossible for us to progress.' He said his and Nigel's names had been 'unfortunately and unjustifiably' tarnished by the affair, and he insisted that Longcare had provided a good standard of care. Both he and Nigel, he said, had decided to leave the care profession for good.

Every former employee I spoke to remains adamant that Ray

Cradock and Nigel Rowe both knew of a number of instances of what was going on.

Debbie said: 'I reported it to Ray Cradock more than once when he was working as a consultant. It was no good taking it to Nigel. He didn't want to know. I think he just shut his eyes. Two weeks after I started, I told Ray about how Gordon had kicked Jackie G. He knew about the physical abuse, because I told him. I also told him that David had been hit because he was supposed to have been "misbehaving" in the garden, and how Gordon had taken David behind the bushes to be punished. I couldn't have been the only one. But somehow, whenever I told him something, it always seemed to get back to Gordon. That was why in the end I stopped telling him these things.'

Another former Longcare employee remembers Cradock interviewing every member of staff to try to find out why morale was so low. 'Every time somebody came up to him with a complaint, he would say, 'Can you put up with it a bit longer, because it won't be long before Gordon retires?' And Nigel used to say, "You know what my dad's like, but he won't be here for much longer."'

The apparent failure of Ray Cradock and Nigel Rowe to act on the complaints only served to underline to their staff how hopeless it was to try to force the authorities to take notice of the allegations, but it also had a more subtle effect. The care workers saw that Nigel and Ray didn't seem to do anything about the abuse, or didn't think it necessary to do anything, and they followed their examples. After all, they were in charge. They should know.

Whether through ignorance, naivety or fear, those employees who had not acted to halt the Longcare regime *had* been guilty—of failing to treat the people they were caring for as their equals, as human beings.

25. Buckinghamshire County Council

> 'However, when we moved to Buckinghamshire I came up against the postcode lottery. Their social services department has offered far less support than Hertfordshire. Our new social worker said the council 'didn't have a big enough purse… Buckinghamshire Council is poorly funded and under-staffed, and parents face long delays in getting

replies to queries about their learning disabled children. The local carers' organisation tells me my plight is all-too familiar.'

Jane Gregory, *Community Care*, December 21, 2000

It must have taken only a couple of seconds, but the signature that a senior Buckinghamshire County Council officer placed upon the document that allowed Gordon Rowe to open a residential home at Stoke Place Mansion House in 1983 was to have devastating consequences.

Eleven years later, the council would admit that it had known Rowe had been investigated by the police in Somerset. The council also admitted that neither Stan Bristow, its principal residential services officer (who approved the registration) nor any of his colleagues, had investigated the claims, or had gone to visit Somerset to test the weight of evidence.

But this was to be only the first in a series of blunders by the council.

Rowe had applied to be the owner and manager of Stoke Place in February, 1983. He told Bucks that he was currently the manager of a home in Somerset and wanted to bring some of its residents and staff with him.

The law demanded that a home manager should be a 'fit and proper person' to be looking after vulnerable adults. If it wished to turn him down, the onus was on the council to prove that Gordon Rowe was unfit to take such a role, and not on him to prove he was suitable. But, crucially, if the council believed he was 'unfit', it would only have to prove so 'on the balance of probabilities'. Evidence of abuse from just one of Rowe's victims in Somerset should have been enough to halt his application.

Rowe provided his four glowing references and, by the end of September, had been told by Bristow what he would need to do to bring Stoke Place up to the required standard. But he had also been told—in advance of the council granting registration—that he could begin telling local authorities that in a month's time the home could start taking in clients. Tom Burgner, who in 1997 was to lead an independent inquiry into the council's handling of the case, told me this was definitely 'bad practice' and had compromised Bristow's position. 'It should not have happened,' he said.

As mentioned above, in October 1983 the Somerset police investigation ended. Both David Fineberg, the owner of The Old Rectory, and Michael Brown, Rowe's successor there, contacted Buckinghamshire

County Council. So, too, did an officer from Somerset County Council and one of the Somerset police officers. Rowe told Bristow he had been set up in a bid to stop him taking residents from The Old Rectory to his new home.

A visit to Somerset would have provided sufficient evidence to prove to Bucks 'on the balance of probabilities' that Gordon Rowe was unfit to be running a home. But that visit was not made, whether through arrogance, through incompetence, through over-work, or because Stan Bristow had told Rowe he would be able to open his home and was fearful of the legal consequences if he changed his mind.

Bristow had left himself no room for manoeuvre and the certificate of registration was issued on November 28, 1983. Eighteen days later, a letter arrived at Bucks social services from the director of social services for the Royal Borough of Kensington and Chelsea. It expressed concern about Rowe and enclosed a copy of a letter written by Michael Brown, in which he said he was '100 per cent convinced of the truth' of the allegations that Rowe had sexually assaulted more than one resident at The Old Rectory. Yet, no attempt was made to investigate the claims.

Years later, the council would defend the decision to register Stoke Place by claiming the police had told them there was no evidence against Rowe. But a Somerset police source insisted that what the council had actually been told was that the investigation *had* produced evidence against Rowe, but that there just hadn't been enough to prove a criminal case beyond all reasonable doubt in court.

I spoke to Stan Bristow early in 1996. Now retired, he was prepared to talk briefly about his role as principal residential services officer for Buckinghamshire in the early 80s.

At the time Rowe applied to register Stoke Place, there were about forty homes in Bristow's remit and he was directly responsible to the director of social services. He told me the council was 'well ahead' of other local authorities in its arrangements for registering and inspecting residential homes.

Bristow was not prepared to talk in depth about why he allowed Rowe to open the home, but he told me: 'I take full responsibility. I care about people and that was it.' If he was inspecting or opening that home at that time, things must have been in his eyes correct, he said because otherwise it would never have been opened, and it would never have been allowed to run.

In fact, Bristow said, Stoke Place was one of a handful of homes he took a particular interest in, joining staff meetings and occasionally calling in 'on the off-chance'. He would visit Stoke Place about once every six to eight weeks, spending a whole day there each time. He said he spent a lot of time with the residents and even attended social events in the evenings. His frequent visits, most of which Rowe would have been aware of in advance, may have been due to his concern over the Somerset allegations, but Bristow wouldn't comment on this.

'If there had been anything untoward going on during my reign, I would have sussed it and I would have done something about it,' he told me. He was adamant that his department was not short-staffed, and said another officer was appointed soon afterwards to work under him.

Gus Gray, the equivalent officer to Bristow with neighbouring Berkshire County Council, has a different story. In 1985, two years after he had been granted permission to open Stoke Place, Gordon Rowe approached Gray for permission to open a large residential home for learning disabled adults on the site of a former boarding school in west Berkshire.

Gray's department had recently written a document concluding that no home for more than sixteen residents would be acceptable to Berkshire. Rowe told Gray and a colleague that he was sure they could 'find a way round the regulations'. He also implied he had connections and would make things unpleasant for them if they did not register him. They warned their boss and submitted a report. Then Rowe contacted them again and was even more abusive. He said they would 'live to regret it'.

Gray believes the registration and inspection department in Buckinghamshire was seriously under-staffed. In Berkshire, there were four inspectors reporting to him, contrasting with one or two staff in total in Bucks.

Gray is convinced his department would never have allowed Rowe to open a home if it had been told about the police investigation in Somerset. But he has a partial explanation for why Bucks allowed Rowe to open Stoke Place. 'Their preparatory work was much less thorough in Bucks and I do not think that agreed registration conditions were stuck to anything like as rigidly as they were in Berkshire,' he told me. Gray believes Bristow was probably having difficulty keeping up-to-date with his formal inspections, and had no time to carry out the vital surprise inspections. 'From what I know, Bristow did not get a lot of support from his superiors, so I think Bucks social services must take some responsibility for what happened.'

Jenny Sleight, a senior Bucks County Council press officer, told me in 1998 that it was 'difficult' to say how many inspectors worked in Buckinghamshire in 1983. 'The actual business of inspection of homes in the county was part of the job of various managers,' she said. This contrasted with the view of Gus Gray, and indeed Stan Bristow, who seemed to have been under the impression that *he* had been the council's specialist inspection and registration officer.

It wasn't for another five years, just before the victim's case against the council was about to commence at the High Court, that I discovered yet another damning piece of evidence that pointed to Buckinghamshire's failure to protect the Longcare residents.

I was told that, on November 21, 1984, almost exactly a year after the council had officially registered Stoke Place as a residential home, a social worker had contacted Stan Bristow with concerns about the home, and Gordon Rowe.

Peter Costello, who worked for the London borough of Hounslow, told Bristow that Gordon Rowe had physically assaulted one of the male residents. He also told him that this resident was not receiving his pocket money and was being punished for coming down late for breakfast. There was, said Costello, an atmosphere of 'apathy and lethargy' about the home, which he believed was short-staffed.

It is not known what action the council took after Costello handed them this information, or whether the allegations were even investigated, but its leaked report, nearly ten years later, made no reference to Costello's concerns. This was at the very least surprising, because these were just the sort of incidents that would be described by the council's inspectors in their 1994 report.

In 1987, Bucks County Council made a further decision in Rowe's favour.

Early the previous year, Rowe had submitted an application to register Stoke Green House as a residential home. Members of the county council's senior management group decided this would mean a large number of learning disabled people concentrated in a small area, and rejected the application.

But Rowe didn't give up. In April, he wrote again to Bucks and persuaded a representative of Slough Mencap to write to South Bucks District Council in support of his planning application to convert Stoke Green House into a residential home. The charity said there was a shortage of residential placements for 'mentally handicapped' people, and until there were enough smaller units, such large homes were filling a need not being met by local authorities.

In April 1987, the director of Bucks social services wrote to the district council to say that they had changed their mind. Although they still had reservations, they registered Gordon and Angela Rowe to run Stoke Green House.

The subsequent Independent Longcare Inquiry of 1997-98 concluded: 'There was [now] a large number of vulnerable adults, in a relatively closed environment, under the control of one man against whom allegations questioning fitness had been made.' There was also no attempt to ensure that the residents would be involved in the community or with outside agencies.

Again, Buckinghamshire had given Gordon Rowe the benefit of the doubt. This, though, was far from the end of the council's failures.

Following Dorothy Abbot's initial claims of abuse by Rowe of April 1991, the council received another complaint. Early in December, 1992, an ex-member of staff called the council anonymously and spoke to the head of the inspection unit, Jennifer Waldron. She said Gordon Rowe was punishing residents by sending them into the garden to eat their breakfast, had kicked a resident on the bottom and 'ordered cold showers'. Two care assistants had told her that Rowe was sexually abusing residents.

Three days later, she called the unit and repeated the allegations, this time giving enough information to be identified. The inspection unit decided that the risk to the residents was 'not one of immediacy', although it did inform the police's family protection unit.

The following day, December 11, the unit received a third telephone call, probably from the same caller. New allegations were added, including further examples of abuse, neglect and ill-treatment.

On December 14, a police officer told Waldron there was not enough witness information to proceed with a criminal inquiry. The inspection unit decided not to make a surprise inspection visit to Longcare, in case they 'tipped off' Gordon Rowe. Instead, they decided to review the situation the following month.

When they met on January 8, the unit decided that if they visited the homes unannounced during the day they would be unlikely to meet many residents. But a visit 'out of hours' would alert the directors. So they decided to continue with an inspection already arranged for February 23, and announce that out of hours visits would be starting across the county, especially in homes for learning disabled people.

The following month, a second caller contacted the inspection unit and gave her name. She stated that a resident had been sent to bed for three to seven days for 'confrontational behaviour'. Staff were encouraged to write in the report book that he was 'unwell, again'.

A week later, on February 23, a third caller provided information about physical assaults, financial irregularities, and insufficient staff. Although he declined to leave his name, he also provided enough information to be identified. Yet again, the unit did not act.

On March 29, four days after a pre-announced inspection had taken place, Allan wrote to Berkshire County Council. His letter was passed on to Bucks. It made allegations of physical and emotional abuse by Gordon and Angela Rowe, including claims that Gordon Rowe had forced Jackie to eat her meals outside on her birthday. When her brother called to wish her happy birthday, he wrote, Gordon Rowe instructed a member of staff not to pass the message on. Allan said Rowe had punched a resident in the face for defecating in his bed and put another man outside to dry his clothes when he wet himself. There was a string of other allegations, including a concern about the length of time Gordon Rowe had spent in a female resident's bedroom after she asked him to kiss her goodnight. Allan said he was willing for his name to be used.

On May 11, the county council issued new registration certificates for Stoke Place and Stoke Green, in the name of Longcare Ltd, and under the management of Ray Cradock. The applications had been made the previous September, but the decision to allow the names of Gordon and Angela Rowe to be removed from the certificates was another serious error. It meant that, because Gordon Rowe was no longer officially in charge, it would be much harder to take action to close the homes. The certificates were also issued without asking Cradock whether he had been aware of any allegations of abuse against Gordon Rowe.

Again and again, the county council had failed to investigate serious allegations of abuse, even though the inspection unit had the power to enter Stoke Place and Stoke Green and probe them in depth. Yet again, the opportunity to protect and supervise the care of the residents of the Longcare homes was passed over.

On July 15, another witness, a former care assistant and friend of Clare Johnson, contacted the council and made serious allegations.

The following day, Slough police agreed to take part in a joint investigation with the inspection unit. It lasted three months, during which time detectives merely took statements from Clare and the two other witnesses who had given their names to the inspection unit. The three telephone callers were not tracked down.

In mid-October, the police told the council there was no-one further they could interview without alerting Gordon Rowe. They also stressed how difficult it was to secure prosecutions in cases involving learning disabled people, and told the inspection unit there was nothing they could do without further evidence.

On November 1, the inspection unit met with Jean Jeffrey, Buckinghamshire's director of social services, to discuss the case. It was now that Bucks finally decided to launch a full investigation. On November 16, Waldron wrote to every local authority known to have a client at Longcare, saying the department was investigating 'several complaints' about the care of residents.

The investigation team took seventeen written statements, which included more than one hundred and forty allegations, involving fifty one residents, stretching from 1988 to late 1993.

There was evidence of physical assaults by Gordon Rowe against more than a dozen residents, including punches, slaps, hosing down with cold water, holding a snooker cue around the neck of a resident and tying another to a tree. There were allegations of punishments, such as sending people to their rooms for days on end, being made to eat meals outside and being forced to sit apart from other residents. There was also evidence that Gordon Rowe had raped his female 'favourites'. Staffing levels, fraud, the exploitation of the 'working lads', inadequate clothing and toiletries, and problems with over-medication were also mentioned, including a series of allegations against Angela Rowe and Lorraine Field. Witnesses had described how Field hit one resident around the head, failed to act when residents were sick, sent one man to bed as a punishment and chased another male resident into the garden. According to the report, one man confided to a member of staff that he was 'scared about upsetting Lorraine and making her angry; he wept, recalling one incident where she had hit him'.

The report's recommendations included requirements that Gordon and Angela Rowe and Lorraine Field should be forbidden from having any involvement with the company or contact with the residents, that the residents should undertake assertiveness training, that there should be more inspection visits, and that staff training should be improved.

'It is difficult,' wrote Waldron, 'to distil the information given and still convey the enormity and scale of humiliation, deprivation, torment and punishment to which residents were subjected.'

But it was not enough. For one thing, Gordon Rowe's name was no longer on the registration documents, so if it wanted to close the homes, the inspection unit would have to prove that Ray Cradock and Nigel Rowe had known the abuse was going on and did nothing to stop it.

A draft report concluded: 'It is impossible but to conclude that all three directors (Angela and Nigel Rowe and Ray Cradock) must have been aware of the repressive nature of the regime which prevailed and by inaction, share the responsibility for its continued existence.' They added: '...the inspection unit's continuing concern is lack of confidence in the owners and manager's ability to protect the residents from the degradation which, on the balance of probabilities, they have suffered in the past.'

On reading the draft report, though, the council's barrister became concerned. He had originally been told that Nigel Rowe and Ray Cradock had probably done all they could to protect residents. Now, following detailed examination of the homes' report books, inspectors were telling him that the two men were almost certainly unfit to be in charge. The barrister asked for more proof.

But the director of Buckinghamshire's social services, was becoming increasingly impatient. She told Waldron to wrap up the investigation and prepare a final report.

In the absence of the necessary proof that Nigel Rowe and Ray Cradock had known what was going on at Longcare, the barrister amended the draft report. There was, he was forced to conclude, insufficient evidence to force the closure of the home. The report now stated that 'Nigel Rowe and Ray Cradock are and were honourable men and decent men who found themselves in a position not of their choosing and in which they were for all practical purposes powerless to act against Gordon Rowe... they are seen as forces for good'.

When members of the council's casework sub-committee met to discuss the report on July 8, 1994, they were handed a file containing a mountain of information, including the inspection unit's report and Longcare's lengthy response. The councillors were not given the chance to read the report in advance. Only the two Labour members argued that the homes should be closed; the others accepted the recommendations suggested by

Jean Jeffrey. At the end of the meeting, the councillors had to hand all the papers back to the officers.

Audrey Bainbridge, the Conservative councillor who chaired the sub-committee, refused to be interviewed for this book, after taking advice from the council's legal department. But Pam Crawford, a Liberal Democrat member of the sub-committee, agreed to discuss what went on.

Crawford said she and her colleagues had discussed the report in detail and 'asked a lot of questions', but were told it was 'not our duty to bring retribution'. She said a major factor in the decision not to close the homes was the shortage of suitable places in other residential homes. A secondary concern was the fear of being sued by Longcare. 'There was no certainty that we would have been able to prove the case. It was our social services that had the concerns—no-one else's. If we had lost the lawsuit, that money would have had to have been paid for by our social services budget,' she told me.

'The other consideration was that once the inspection had got underway, the Rowes had distanced themselves. It was the Rowes who were the real culprits and therefore without them being there the danger was more or less gone. We asked a lot of questions about the son. We had no complaints about his behaviour and there was some evidence that on one or two occasions he had intervened.'

Labour councillor Trevor Fowler also spoke to me about the meeting. He was to discover later that Jean Jeffrey and her officers had not been 'totally straight' with him and his colleagues. 'There was revulsion and sickness on my part on reading the detail that was put in there, and I suspect other members felt the same as well. The real difference was in what do we do about it.' He and Labour colleague Dick O'Brien argued for closure, but were easily out-voted by the Conservative and Liberal Democrat majority. The report was sent to the local authorities with residents at the homes on July 20, along with a copy of Longcare's comments. It was forwarded to Thames Valley Police on August 11. Just over a week later, Bucks met representatives of the sponsoring authorities and passed on specific information about particular residents.

Four weeks after we published our first Longcare story, the *Slough Observer* had reported that Bucks investigators were given evidence that Nigel Rowe and Ray Cradock knew of allegations that Gordon Rowe had abused residents. Yet the previous week Jean Jeffrey told a meeting of the social services committee that her department had carried out a 'massive search' of the homes' records and failed to unearth any evidence that the two men were unfit to be running the homes.

The county councillors who made the decision to allow the Longcare homes to stay open were not told two vital facts. First that the inspectors themselves believed that both Cradock and Nigel Rowe had known for several years about certain aspects of Gordon Rowe's brutal regime. Secondly, that although the council's barrister had recommended that the inspection unit should seek extra evidence about the fitness of Cradock and Nigel Rowe, Jean Jeffrey had told the inspection unit not to do this because they had run out of time.

It was only four years later, with the publication of the Longcare Inquiry report, that the *Slough Observer* and the two Labour councillors were proved right. Fowler told me: 'One of the things the inquiry report showed was that there was a strong feeling within the inspection department that de-registration should take place, but we were never told that the inspection unit took that view. I have never felt so strongly that a view that I have held has been vindicated.'

Tom Burgner, the head of the Independent Longcare Inquiry that was ordered by Parliamentary Under Secretary of State Paul Boateng, concluded in 1998, at the end of nine months, that the county council had made 'serious mistakes', although lessons had since been learned. He made 95 separate recommendations, most of which were directed at Bucks. But there were also key messages for the government.

The Independent Longcare Inquiry delivered a trenchant criticism of the county council's investigation. It concluded that its work had been unfocussed and tentative. It said the inspection unit had waited far too long to obtain evidence from the report books, and then failed to develop that line of enquiry. Crucially, it failed to interview residents and therefore was not able to determine whether they were at risk. The inspectors also failed to talk to social workers and relatives, or talk to experts who could have decided whether the residents would be seriously at risk if the homes stayed open.

Although highly critical of the council in his report, Burgner did feel there had been mitigating circumstances, he told me. 'Gordon Rowe obviously cultivated people he thought would be useful in the police, and possibly elsewhere, too. I think I would accept that his success in making himself to some extent a pillar of the community made life particularly difficult for the inspection unit team. They were dealing with someone who was influential in the community.'

Yet the council's final report, the inquiry concluded, did not reflect the inspectors' view that the homes should be closed. Their investigation stopped 'just as it began to focus on the supporting information it needed' to show that the homes should be shut and that Nigel Rowe and Ray Cradock were unfit to be running residential homes.

The inquiry also found that information about the allegations should have been passed on much sooner to the local authorities that had placed clients in the homes. They had only been given details of the allegations at the end of July, 1994. This delay meant that the families of the residents also had no idea what had been alleged, and allowed their loved ones to continue living at Longcare for much longer than was necessary.

Neither Jean Jeffrey, Jennifer Waldron, nor Audrey Bainbridge were present at the press conference held by the county council on the day the Independent Longcare Inquiry report was published in June, 1998. Waldron was no longer in her post, although it was unclear whether she had left permanently or was on sick leave. Bainbridge had been promoted to deputy leader of the council's Conservative group. And on the very day the report was published, the council announced that Jeffrey was leaving after more than seven years service.

Jeffrey's own press release was congratulatory. Indeed, some members of the press wondered whether she had been handed the wrong inquiry report. 'The Burgner report shows that we took reasonable action in 1994, and recognises the determination and success of the inspection unit and of Thames Valley Police in pursuing the protection of people, within the constraints of the legislation in place at the time,' she announced. That was quite definitely not the conclusion reached by Burgner and his colleagues, who had heavily criticised her decision to stop the investigation just as it was about to find the evidence it needed to close the two homes.'

'The senior officers and senior management of the council were privy to what the report contained [before it was published] and they chose not to lose one minute,' Trevor Fowler told me. 'They acted to make sure that when the report was actually published, Jean Jeffrey was not there. Everyone knew that she had gone because of Longcare.'

But Fowler also believed the county councillors on the ruling Conservative group had got off lightly. 'Nothing stuck to the politicians and yet they had made the final decisions about these things,' he said.

The council itself accepted the findings of the inquiry and that the inspection unit had made mistakes. 'We are deeply sorry for this and apologise to the residents and their families,' it stated in a press release.

Abuse of any kind is easier to detect—and deter—when systems are in place to allow the free flow of information between all the parties concerned, be they residents, care workers, social workers, inspectors, police officers or relatives. Communication is vital. Once a robust system is in place which encourages communication, then those responsible have only two further tasks: to listen and to act—immediately, and with vigour and determination. Buckinghamshire failed in all of these tasks, and in so doing failed the residents of Longcare, and needlessly exposed them to years of cruelty, neglect and misery.

26. The Police

> 'When Stephen Downing walked free yesterday after serving 27 years for a crime he probably never committed, it was not startling new evidence that cleared his path... it was a procedural travesty that gave him his liberty... When Mr Downing was arrested in September 1973 for the murder of Wendy Sewell, he was questioned from 2.30pm until 11pm before being charged. He was not cautioned until 10.30pm and, according to police statements still in existence, he appears never to have been told he was entitled to see a solicitor. According to Julian Bevan QC, representing the Crown at the Court of Appeal yesterday, there is reason to believe Mr Downing, then a 17-year-old with a mental age of 11, asked for a solicitor but was denied access to one.'
>
> *The Independent*, February 8, 2001

It was September 1994, and the Longcare case was rapidly proving a particular embarrassment to Thames Valley Police, which had twice failed to properly investigate claims of sexual abuse, ill-treatment, neglect and assault against Gordon Rowe.

The council's inspection unit had gathered a wealth of evidence, without interviewing a single alleged victim. It didn't take long for the force to acknowledge—at least internally—that something had gone badly wrong.

Within hours of the publication of the story in the *Slough Observer* and *The Independent*, other newspapers, radio and television stations were following it up. Questions were being asked about Rowe's close relationship with certain police officers. Chief Constable Charles Pollard decided something had to be done. He ordered a new investigation to be launched immediately, under the title of Operation Skip.

The officer Pollard chose to lead the investigation was Detective Superintendent Jon Bound. Bound's CV boasted a string of high-profile investigations. He intended to retire from the force in little more than a year and this was to be his last big case. He was also squeaky clean and had no links with Slough police.

Within hours of reviewing the case, Bound concluded that Slough had not dealt with the case properly, for whatever reason. He realised that— because of the media pressure—his investigation would need to be faultless and exhaustive. In his opinion, Longcare was 'a sore that was not going to go away'.

On Thursday, September 23, police officers raided Stoke Place Mansion House, Rowe's cottage in the grounds of Stoke Place, Stoke Green House, and Rowe's home in Windsor. They removed a mass of evidence from 12 Harrington Close, including several large crates of documents, boxes of videotapes and a police helmet belonging to one of Rowe's friends.

Thames Valley Police's first official, documented involvement with Longcare had occurred late in 1992, when Slough's family protection unit was told about the allegations made anonymously to the inspection unit. It had also been given details of Rowe's 1991 assault on Dorothy Abbott. A police officer made it clear to the council that they could not take the matter forward without a formal complaint, but agreed to read the files.

After the third anonymous telephone call, Waldron and the council inspector responsible for the Longcare homes met with a sergeant from the family protection unit to discuss the allegations. He told them there was not enough evidence to proceed with a criminal investigation.

Six months later, following allegations from four more former members of Longcare staff, Slough police finally launched an investigation, supposedly in collaboration with the inspection unit. It lasted about two months, but consisted only of interviewing members of staff who had made complaints, including Clare, who had come forward on July 15. The detectives' superior, a detective inspector, was later to tell the Longcare inquiry: 'At this stage it was felt that the management of the homes should not be made aware of the enquiry and that the investigators should concentrate on interviewing ex-members of staff, or any people who were unlikely to inform Gordon Rowe or the management of the homes of our enquiries. This was to ensure, as far as possible, that should a full investigation take place, no evidence would be lost. The enquiry was not to be made general knowledge to other police officers at Slough.'

This final sentence was a clear acknowledgement of the close personal relationships that Gordon Rowe had formed with a number of Slough police officers.

But the inquiries was almost immediately scaled down when both the officers were drafted in to the incident room of an investigation into the murder of a little boy, Aklaq Ahmed, whose body had been found in a park near his family's Slough home. The Longcare file was reallocated to another detective constable, who again was chosen because he had no connection to Gordon Rowe.

By early October 1993, the new detective had taken statements from just two witnesses and the inspection unit were becoming increasingly frustrated. On October 7, Waldron wrote to the detective inspector heading the inquiry and said she believed residents were still being subjected to serious abuse and that her unit was having problems contacting the officer on the case.

A week later, the detective inspector met with one of his superiors, a detective superintendent, to discuss the evidence. The DI contacted the Crown Prosecution Service (CPS) informally, and was told there was nothing it could do without the full papers and further evidence. The CPS was never asked for a formal opinion.

The detective inspector, detective sergeant and detective constable met with Waldron and four other council officers on October 14. They said there was nobody else they could interview without alerting Gordon Rowe, that the evidence of learning disabled people was difficult to use in court, and that the investigation in 1983 in Somerset had also proved fruitless. They handed the case back to the inspection unit.

It was not until August 12, 1994, nearly 12 months later, when they received a copy of the inspection unit's report, that Thames Valley Police heard more about the Longcare case. Even then, no action was taken until the first stories appeared in the press on September 16, 1994.

Whatever had happened in the past, Supt Jon Bound was now taking the allegations seriously. His first step was to bring together a team of four police officers, three of whom had backgrounds in family protection work and often dealt with sexually abused children. But none of the quartet, or Bound himself, had any experience or training in interviewing learning disabled people.

As with the two previous investigations, none of Bound's team had any links with Gordon Rowe or the Freemasons, and only the members of this small team were allowed access to the case computer files.

Bound set up his incident room at Langley police station, a couple of miles from the gates of Stoke Place. His strategy was simple: to interview every current and former member of staff who had worked at the two homes since 1987. It was to take more than 12 months.

They began tracing former members of staff. A confidential hotline advertised in the Press produced many of the names. They also researched the issues surrounding people with learning difficulties: what is Down's syndrome? How are residential homes supposed to be run? How does the complaints system work?

A picture soon began to emerge of the regime Gordon Rowe had instigated. Names of particular residents began to re-occur during different interviews. Some had been victims of particular instances of sexual or physical assaults, others suffered from the general inhumanity of the regime.

The team eventually compiled evidence of forty residents they believed had been subjected to various forms of 'abuse', dating from 1983 to 1994. Forensic psychologists assessed all of the alleged victims to judge their levels of competence. A small number were considered able to give evidence in a court-room. It was an easy victory over the ill-conceived reactions of the police officers in the first two investigations who dismissed the chance of any residents appearing as witnesses.

The evidence was there. It had always been there, if only the police had come looking for it. Bound told me: 'It was quite clear that there was a considerable amount of physical and sexual abuse. It was also clear that Gordon Rowe had been having sexual intercourse with the prettier female residents. The majority of physical abuse was whacking around the back of the head and kicking up the backside, where there were no injuries.'

This created a problem. With no evidence of injuries, there was little chance of achieving convictions for physical assaults. Bound realised the only option was to resort to the 40-year-old Mental Health Act, and prosecute the perpetrators for ill-treatment and neglect of 'mentally disordered patients'. The wording was another throwback to the days of the Victorian asylums, but it was the best the British legal system could offer.

As for the sexual charges, Bound knew that, because there were few if any other witnesses, and only circumstantial evidence, the victims themselves would have to give evidence in court.

Towards the end of 1995, the police team were left with allegations against 15 current and former members of Longcare staff, including Gordon and Angela Rowe, Desmond Tully and Lorraine Field. Each was interviewed, but none of them admitted a single offence. In November, the 14-month investigation ended and thousands of pages of police evidence were sent to the Crown Prosecution Service. The team had interviewed 800 people, taken 519 statements and collated 1,178 documents.

But although Thames Valley Police had finally succeeded in investigating most of the allegations against Gordon Rowe and his sidekicks—relatives of the victims believe that the allegations of fraud were never satisfactorily probed—its problems were far from over.

Bound had been so concerned at the apparent links between Rowe and Slough police that, at the start of his investigation, he notified the Police Complaints Authority (PCA), which agreed to oversee an internal inquiry by the force's own complaints and discipline department.

For years, Rowe had used his links with the force, and Slough police station in particular, to intimidate both residents and staff, and to ensure they knew that complaints made against him would be dismissed out of hand. Officers from Slough police were frequent social visitors to Stoke Place, Rowe leant them one of the Longcare minibuses for fishing trips, and a former care worker claimed a detective had told her that nobody from Slough police would take on the case because it involved Gordon Rowe.

None of this was proof of anything, but given the two police investigations that had been abandoned, the suspicions were clear.

When the 18-month internal investigation ended, in January 1998, it concluded that the allegations against Rowe had not been adequately dealt with in the first two investigations. A PCA spokesman told me: 'There was no evidence to suggest that officers neglected their duties, but, clearly, inappropriate decisions were taken. There were various accusations made which should have been investigated earlier.'

The PCA's report mentioned two police officers, Officer A and Officer B—neither of whose names were made public. Among the most serious of the accusations levelled at the two men was that residents were taken by Rowe on several occasions to both of their homes to carry out decorating and landscaping work for little or no money. The inquiry also found that Officer A had used the force's national computer to carry out checks on the criminal records of members of Rowe's staff. And it discovered evidence that Rowe had invited this officer to Stoke Place on at least four occasions, to deliver 'warnings' to residents about their behaviour.

The PCA spokesman said: 'These were people who were very susceptible and very vulnerable and would obviously feel very threatened by police officers coming in and warning them. It was inappropriate and it is very doubtful that these warnings were given as part of the carrying out of their statutory duties.'

The internal investigation was fraught with difficulties. Most of the witnesses were learning disabled people and so, the PCA said, the allegations could not be proved to a degree sufficient to bring any formal disciplinary charges. Instead, the two men were handed 'admonishments', temporary black marks entered on a police officer's disciplinary record, usually only for 12 months.

No-one at Thames Valley Police was prepared to discuss the internal inquiry with me. I was told it was 'confidential'.

The force eventually sent me a copy of a 'protocol' developed with the county council, a direct result of the Longcare case, said a spokesman. 'There was a lot of discussion after the inquiries finished, asking what did we do wrong? What could we do? Were we as good as we could have been? [The answer was] no we were not.'

The *Joint Protocol for Investigations of Abuse of Vulnerable Adults in Buckinghamshire* is a worthy document and would probably have led to concerted action being taken sooner if it had been in place in 1992. It provides guidelines on how to respond to an initial allegation of abuse, how to proceed with an investigation, how to set up and run a joint investigation with social services departments or health authorities, and how to plan for court proceedings.

Although the third police investigation had been carried out with determination and the full backing of the force, the officers involved had still lacked detailed knowledge of how to investigate allegations of abuse of learning disabled people. They learned as they went along, but at least they tried.

The question remains, though: why were Slough police initially so reluctant to launch a full investigation into the allegations against Gordon Rowe?

There were several reasons: Rowe's close relationship with Slough police and his 'reputation' in the community, the reluctance of the officers involved in the first two investigations to make any effort to understand learning disabled people, and the failure of the English legal system to protect vulnerable adults.

27. Gordon Rowe

'A retired French bus driver has admitted murdering seven young, mentally handicapped women in the 70s but he may never be tried for his crimes. The confession of Emile Louis, 66—after three years of denials—turns him overnight into one of the worst serial killers in French history... The case has revealed more than two decades of indifference, cover-ups and bungling by the French welfare and judicial systems.'

The Independent, December 16, 2000

Gordon's sister, Maureen, once confided to a member of Longcare staff that she believed her brother was mentally ill. She couldn't find any other explanation for his behaviour. 'I can remember days when Gordon wasn't like this. On family holidays, when we were younger, Gordon would always have people with mental handicaps around him,' she said. 'He used to round them up like a sheepdog. When he opened his first home in Somerset, it was like a lifelong ambition for him—he was such a caring person. And when he opened Longcare, he brought all the family along and told them he wanted it to be a happy home and he wanted us all to work there.'

Maureen—who didn't know then about the allegations from The Old Rectory, and, even earlier, from Sussex—believed money and power changed her brother. Gordon pushed his family away as the cash flooded in. His brother Ted was forced to take legal action to recover money he invested in Longcare. In the end, he is said to have received £14,000 and a new car.

Many of the staff knew about the residents' holiday at Butlin's, when

Gordon had locked himself in the bathroom for three days. Ted told one care assistant he believed his brother had had a breakdown and never recovered.

But explaining why Rowe did what he did is not as easy as that. He was abusing children—and probably people with learning difficulties—as early as 1969, and maybe even earlier. Was there something in his past that could explain his need for sexual domination over vulnerable people? Or was he just possessed of a monumental ego and a sadistic disregard for others? Was he, in fact, a psychopath?

A letter Gordon Rowe wrote to a neighbour in Harrington Close nearly four months after the abuse was exposed provides the clearest evidence of his mental state at the time.

He described how he and his family had returned home after three months away, 'following the horrific allegations so luridly and sensationally printed in the local and national Press'.

'There is a completely contradictory story to this situation but, right from the start, we were told to "shut up" and "make no comment whatsoever" and, thus, we have been unable to put our side of things,' he wrote. 'Certainly, our "absence" and "silence" implies guilt to most people but our legal advisers told us—and we firmly believe it—that the Press would *not* have published anything that was contrary to the story that they had told or of the image that they had portrayed of us.'

He claimed none of the allegations had been witnessed by a second person and that if something had been going on, the care workers who left Longcare would have reported them to the authorities. He also denied intimidating his employees.

'Considerable "contra-evidence" has been submitted to the Police but it is *still essential at this time* that these facts are not relayed to the Press who will again have a field-day by re-opening their coverage. Our opportunity to hit back will occur on completion of the present Police enquirey [sic],' he wrote.

Rowe had lost none of his cunning. He was trying to portray himself and Angela as innocent victims of a vicious conspiracy. 'I am writing to you and placing my trust in your discretion and integrity *not* to inform the Press, but to give even just one Resident of Harrington Close the firm assurance that they do not have 'monsters in their midst'. We would dearly love for you to visit us to hear (and see) the other side of this appalling story after which, we feel sure, we may receive a little support that we so desperately need.

'We are living in a nightmare—curtains drawn, lights out, etc, and we are not certain what sort of any long-term effect it may have on Ben who we had to take out of school for the whole of last term. His Headmaster, fortunately, has been 100 per cent supportive and has seen, he says, the same thing happen to Teachers as is happening to us.'

Tuesday, February 21, 1995. Harrington Close, Windsor.

I pulled up alongside the kerb and looked across the road at the large, detached, red-brick house. The graffiti had been cleaned from the large French window. All the curtains were drawn.

For so long, Gordon Rowe had been merely a shadowy form, described second-hand by people who knew him. There were so many unanswered questions. Did he really believe he was innocent? Why had he done what he had done? And how would he behave when confronted?

I walked across the road, up the tarmac driveway and along the path to Rowe's front door. I knocked twice. After a couple of seconds, there were footsteps. The door opened. The squat, white-haired figure of Gordon Rowe was standing in the doorway, wearing an open-necked shirt and blue sweater. For a couple of seconds, my mind went blank.

'Mr Rowe, I'm from the *Slough Observer*. I wonder if....'

'Oh, no, no...'

The door slammed shut.

'Mr Rowe, have you got any comment about the serious allegations you're facing?'

That was my second and final interview with Gordon Rowe.

Six months later, Rowe tried to kill himself. The previous day, August 7, he had arrived at Maidenhead police station, confident he could talk his way out of the allegations, as he had done before. But he had a surprise waiting for him.

It was a long-arranged appointment. The police team had spent months investigating his background and interviewing witnesses, and they told Rowe about the thousands of pages of evidence they had compiled.

Madeleine Stewart was one of the officers who interviewed him. She told me: 'Our aim was to interview him in some depth and he indicated that that was what he wanted. We started the first day very slowly and went all through his background, and that took all day. He was polite and articulate, but quite old by this time and, like him or not, he had been through an extremely hard time. He had been hounded from his house, his whole life had been totally devastated, and obviously that had an effect on him.'

After eight hours questioning, he was released again on police bail, ready to continue the interview the next day. But, instead of returning home to Harrington Close, Rowe drove the two hours to Brighton, where he had friends and Angela had family. He stopped on the way to buy a jar of sleeping pills and some alcohol, and checked into a hotel.

Angela was distraught when he failed to return home. The two of them had pledged to carry out a suicide pact if either of them failed to clear their names. She phoned Maidenhead police station in hysterics and said her husband was missing and might have killed himself. A warrant was issued for his arrest.

Gordon Rowe was eventually found in a hotel room with a suicide note and a half-empty bottle of pills by his side. One Sussex police officer later described it as a 'half-hearted attempt to kill himself'. Rowe was arrested and taken to hospital.

He was admitted soon afterwards to the Cardinal Clinic in Windsor for a psychiatric evaluation and daily treatment. Rowe was admitted to Fairmile Hospital in Cholsey, and later transferred to a hospital in Reading for outpatient treatment.

As Rowe continued to receive treatment for 'depression and anxiety', Det Supt Bound made repeated requests, through Rowe's solicitor, to continue the police interview. His psychiatrist repeatedly said he believed he was not fit to be questioned.

Five months later, Rowe tried to kill himself again, this time at home. The police only found out at the subsequent trial of his wife.

Eventually, Bound conceded defeat. Early in March, he rang Rowe's solicitors and told them Gordon and Angela Rowe were to be charged. He also called the solicitors of Desmond Tully and Lorraine Field. Tully, who now ran a successful residential home in Devon, and Field, who worked as a receptionist in Slough, would be charged with ill-treatment and neglect. Angela Rowe would face similar charges, plus one of indecent assault against a male resident.

But most of the charges were against Gordon Rowe, who was to be accused of three rapes, several indecent assaults and several offences of ill-treatment and neglect. Bound said he could have been charged with 'hundreds' of offences. He told Rowe's solicitor that his client should attend Maidenhead police station on Monday, March 18.

*

On the evening of March 17, Gordon and Angela visited Nigel and his family at their new home in Windsor. Nigel would later say that his dad seemed happier than he had for some months. The two of them spent the evening using Nigel's telescope and discussing astronomy. At about 8.30pm, Gordon and Angela returned home to Crowthorne. They stayed up until early the next morning, discussing their life and talking about their grandchildren, Nigel's children. Angela finally went to bed, leaving Gordon alone.

Angela woke the next morning and realised her husband was not next to her in bed. She ran downstairs and into the kitchen. On the table was a note, addressed to her, Nigel and Ben.

A little earlier that morning, at 5.45am, a man walking his dog had seen a Ford Granada parked at the side of Devil's Highway, a rough track that led off one of the main roads into Crowthorne. In the front seat, a stocky, white-haired man sat asleep, his head lolling to one side. The car had been parked back from the track, in a lay-by. As the dog-walker approached the car, he realised the man was slumped against the door, the engine was still running and a limp hose-pipe was dangling through the car window.

Rowe was already dead. The spot he had chosen to kill himself was within sight of the walls of Broadmoor Hospital, and just a few hundred yards from the house in Crowthorne High Street where he and his brothers and sisters had grown up.

I walked up the gravel driveway past Nigel's red Ferrari. The house appeared empty, but I knocked anyway. No reply. I knocked again and peered through the glass panel, but saw nothing but the foggy outline of a hallway. I turned and walked back down the driveway to my car. Just as I was settling into the front seat, a station wagon appeared in my wing mirror. It slowed as it approached the bend, and turned into Nigel Rowe's driveway. Sitting in the front seat was Nigel Rowe.

'Nigel, I wondered if there was anything you would like to say about your father's death,' I said as I approached.

He looked at me for the first time, his face red. We stood ten feet apart. 'You've got a nerve coming here. Leave now. Get out of here.' He stepped a pace towards me.

'I wanted to give you a chance to say something about your father.'

He paused, and there was the crunch of gravel as he rocked slightly back on his heels. He took a breath. 'I'm sorry. It's been a difficult week,' said Nigel. 'I was thinking of releasing some kind of statement to the Press. OK. What I would like to say is that the intense Press pressure had a direct bearing on my father's death.' 'He maintained his innocence in a suicide note. Never once in two years had he ever had one allegation put to him formally, either by Bucks County Council or by Thames Valley Police, and really I think the pressure over the last three years was just intolerable. It was too much to bear. Another thing he referred to was the Dunblane tragedy, and he thinks he is going onto a better world than the one he left behind.'

'He had not been charged with anything, but he did have a pre-arranged meeting planned yesterday with the police. His brother, Ted, died nearly a year ago to the day and he had just buried another brother two weeks ago, the third in 14 months.'

He paused. 'He had been tried and convicted by the press.'

'Have you had any reaction to his death?' I asked.

'Of course, he will be greatly missed. Tributes are pouring in from family and friends. The funeral will be a private affair.' The words kept tumbling out, all the months and years of anger and frustration released. 'He was very rational. The letter was very rational. He was not disturbed and the balance of his mind was not disturbed. A lot of the contributing causes were that for three years he had never once had an allegation put to him. I think it was the intense Press speculation and media attention that had a direct bearing on his death.'

As I wrote the final few words in my notebook, he took three steps forward until he was a foot or so from my face: 'I hope you feel proud of yourself.'

A month after Rowe's death, a few reporters were the only witnesses to his inquest at Windsor Guildhall. There was little evidence read out by coroner Robert Wilson. Wilson only read extracts from the note Angela Rowe had found in her kitchen on the morning of her husband's death:

Monday, March 18, 1.40am.

My dearest Angela, Ben and Nigel,
the fact that I have disappeared and the discovery of this letter will immediately alert you as to what my intentions are and, by the time you read it...

It is a fact that I have been psychiatrically ill. I was first diagnosed last August. For many months and since then I have been receiving in-patient treatment for most of that time. I have been depressed and anxious...

You know well my belief in God and a new life after death and for that reason, and I am sure it has worried you, I do not fear death.

Your ever-loving husband and father,
Gordon.

Wilson said: 'I think he intended to take his own life.'

28. The Other Visitors

'I gave birth to a profoundly disabled girl who was blind with severe learning difficulties and, worst of all, chronic and life-threatening epilepsy... I attend a support group for parents of special needs children. Many issues are discussed, but the one that provokes the most anger is that, in addition to all our other daily battles, we seem to have to fight against the medical profession. It is a struggle that often starts with the manner in which the initial prognosis is broken and continues through the child's life... unless the arrogance of the medical profession is cured, the ills of the NHS will never be eradicated.'

Linnet Macintyre, *The Observer*, January 21, 2001

No matter how hard he tried to create a culture of isolation and secrecy at Longcare, Gordon Rowe could not prevent everyone visiting his two residential homes. For more than 10 years, dentists, nurses, doctors, chiropodists, parents of prospective residents and representatives of voluntary organisations were all passing through the doors. So if Rowe was beating, raping and neglecting his clients, why did these visitors not notice and raise the alarm?

Rowe may have been a vicious bully, but he made sure his visitors never saw that side of his character. The residents were desperate to get into Gordon's books and would never do anything to annoy him in front of a guest—they knew what the consequences would be. It is possible to see how this fearful willingness to please might convince visitors—

especially those with no specialist training—that what they were seeing was a happy, well-run home.

One worker from the voluntary sector visited the homes regularly after Rowe set up his business in 1983. By the time Rowe bought Stoke Green House, four years later, she remembers the London boroughs 'almost snatching his hand off' to take places because the shortage of beds was so acute. 'I could see the pound signs in Gordon's eyes,' she said.

She saw many signs of poor care over the years, but never dreamed he could be responsible for the scale of abuse eventually revealed. On one occasion, she walked into reception to find Rowe with a woman with Down's syndrome on his lap. He was totally unphased, and told her: 'Don't worry; she thinks of me as her daddy.'

'I told him it was totally inappropriate. What worried me was that he didn't think it was wrong,' she said.

On other occasions, she was shocked at the way he spoke to some of the residents. He used to tell them to 'get your fat arse out of here', or 'get out the back, you big fat slob', but again, she thought it was simply poor judgement combined with an unpleasant bullying streak. She sometimes saw Longcare residents in Slough, and, although they were often dirty and poorly dressed, they never gave her grounds for greater concern.

'If I had known there was real physical or sexual abuse I would have done something about it. I just thought it was inappropriate behaviour or bad management. I knew he had a flawed character, but I didn't believe it was anything worse than that.'

Although it is easy to conclude that she should have complained to the authorities, she was hardly the first to be fooled.

Another outsider who often visited Longcare was Slough pharmacist John Ross, who supplied prescription medicines to the homes. When I spoke to him in January, 1998, he told me that he had found Rowe 'a perfectly normal sort of chap, pleasant and polite'. 'The residents all seemed to treat Gordon on a friendly basis, and there was certainly no sign of fear or anything like that. I didn't see a single incident that would make me raise my eyebrows, bearing in mind my job was to deliver medicine to a carer in the home and I was only ever there for five minutes. The first I heard of any problems was when I read about them in the papers. I was shocked when I read about the report.'

Ross says he saw nothing that alarmed him in the quantities of drugs he was asked to supply. 'Mental medicine is a science of its own; they are not normal doses. They were certainly well within tolerances, otherwise I would have queried it. It is difficult for me to comment correctly, because I wasn't familiar with the patients. My responsibility was purely to dispense the medication.'

Despite the huge weight of evidence, Ross cannot bring himself to believe that the Gordon Rowe he knew was guilty of the allegations made against him.

Ross was not the only healthcare professional to support Longcare's work. At a subsequent court hearing, three professionals who regularly visited the homes also denied ever seeing anything 'untoward' at Stoke Place or Stoke Green.

Henryk Cholewa, an optician in Slough, said in a statement: 'The home always struck me as a friendly and well run place. If I had an elderly relative, this is the place I would choose for them to go.'

Community charge nurse and care manager Jeswant Jessy told the court he had been paying quarterly visits to the Longcare homes since 1987 and had never seen anything that disturbed him. The residents, he added, were always clean and appropriately dressed.

Chiropodist Keith Stodgell and his wife treated residents every six weeks between 1983 and 1993. 'My wife and I never noticed anything at all to concern us. Everyone was clean and well presented. It was delightfully happy. I used to enjoy going there. There was a lot of laughter and a lot of fun,' he said.

These statements showed how easy it was for Rowe to fool outsiders into believing he ran a happy, well-managed home, particularly if he knew exactly when they would be visiting.

Many parents of prospective residents also visited the homes, usually to be shown round by Gordon Rowe.

Rowe was hardly likely to let them see anything incriminating, but he never bothered to disguise his beliefs about the right way to care for learning disabled people. One mother remembers him showing her one of the classrooms at Stoke Place. Some of the more disabled residents were there, with little to occupy them but a few beads. Some had even been tied to their chairs. She remembers Rowe saying: 'These are the very disabled. There is not much anyone can do for these.' She was astonished to hear such words from a care home boss.

However, she found Rowe courteous, and he spent a lot of time with her. His sales patter was as good as ever. There were factual elements to what he told her, but these facts were exaggerated and embellished. He lied about the facilities, his plans for expansion, and the social side of life at Longcare.

No first-time visitor to Longcare would be able to see through such lies. Although some of his attitudes may have been disturbing, Rowe was never going to allow such visitors to see the real Longcare.

Theoretically, no outsiders were better placed to see the real Longcare than the Georges. Their club was joined to the home, after all. David George picked up his post from the Stoke Place reception every morning. Staff at the country club would often look out of their windows and see residents on the lawn, and Rowe frequently visited the club.

David George died in August, 1998, and his widow Chris now runs the country club. She remembers that, although they were grateful to Gordon for saving their business, they had to be on their guard. Rowe had told club members he wanted to take over the whole of Stoke Place. He wanted his own club where he could entertain his friends.

David and Chris George frequently spoke to residents, particularly the more able ones like John F and Bob. But nothing they said led them or any of their staff to suspect Gordon or Angela Rowe of abuse. Perhaps they didn't recognise signs of abuse for what they were. Perhaps they were just not close enough to see what the Longcare regime was really like behind its closed doors.

All Chris George knew was that 'the place was a tip. We knew how dirty it was. It seems incredible that you can live next door and not know what was going on, but we knew nothing about it until one of my sons' friends phoned and said his dad had just seen Stoke Place on the news'.

One of the most striking, and important, aspects of the regime was the absence of contact between Longcare residents and their neighbours in Slough and South Bucks. This was particularly noticeable among those who lived in the small homes Gordon Rowe set up in Slough for some of his more able residents.

It was clear from talking to the neighbours of these small homes that they had never spoken to their disabled occupants. This was particularly true of those who lived near Longcare's home in Myrtle Crescent, situated in the middle of a Slough council estate. The residents of Myrtle Crescent saw their neighbours were in some way 'not normal', and kept their distance. But in doing so, they deprived these men and women of the chance to make friends among 'outsiders'. It was these friendships—and the trust they would have engendered—which might have provided an opportunity for a whispered confidence, or the kind of conversation that finally led to Rowe's downfall.

29. The Medical Profession

> '"There is no point working your guts out to help him because he will never be normal."—a comment from a consultant on a child of two.'
>
> Extract from a report on discrimination in the NHS against people with Down's syndrome; Down's Syndrome Association; March, 1999

Of all the outsiders coming to a residential care home for people with learning difficulties, the one who is probably in the best position to spot signs of abuse is the GP. As a well-educated, medically astute figure with regular confidential access to the residents, a GP will have many advantages over regular staff at a home and other less well-trained visitors when it comes to spotting abuse.

Having his ordinary practice with which to contrast unusual patterns of medical symptoms, a GP is in a unique position to be vigilant of suspicious physical symptoms, unusual sexual or sexualised behaviour, or behaviour indicative of untoward stress, exceptional levels of medication and contraception. He will have the medical training to act with authority towards the homes' management if his concern is raised. In addition, he will have his own patient records to refer back to. When GPs are visited by patients, they keep accurate records, including notes of any medication or other treatment. This allows them to keep an accurate medical history for each patient. This is of course no different when the patient happens to have a learning difficulty.

Medical treatment and appropriate levels of medication of people with a learning disability is a specialised area of their care. Even now, however, this aspect of the Longcare regime remains shrouded in mystery. A great many years after the abuse was first exposed, after the police investigation into the abuse, and after the report of the Independent Longcare Inquiry, new developments continue to unfold. It is increasingly clear that a proper expert investigation of these issues has yet to be carried out to set a proper standard of care.

*

One GP visited the Longcare homes once a week. A doctor in his thirties, he had joined a practice local to the homes in August 1990. It would seem that Gordon Rowe soon befriended him. The GP was often to be seen by staff members chatting with Gordon and Angela in the reception of Stoke Place over a coffee, and he was said to be a golfing partner of another member of the Rowe family. In addition, Gordon Rowe took the GP for meals at Blaze's, the Windsor nightclub where he also took favoured staff and residents (paid for with his clients' money, as it later turned out).

The GP seems to have been well placed to exercise his medical duties and command authority with the Rowes. It is, however, not known whether the GP, in fact, brought concerns about abuse or inadequate conditions to the attention of Longcare management. The GP does not seem to have reported such concerns to the authorities.

Some former members of staff at Longcare have expressed criticism about the GP's approach to medical care for the residents. Clare Johnson, now a successful social care officer, remembers watching the GP give contraceptive injections to at least five of Gordon's Girls, one after the other. She says he delivered the jabs in a toilet that led off the main reception area at Stoke Place. 'The girls would come down and basically he would have them pull their trousers down,' she says. She remembers that he continued talking about holiday homes in the USA with Gordon Rowe, who was sitting in reception, while he was delivering the injections. 'The toilet door was still open,' says Clare, and the GP 'was not even talking to the girls, not even acknowledging that they existed.'

The delivering of contraceptive injections was a procedure repeated by the GP every few weeks, says Clare. She worked at Longcare for nearly four years, and says she never saw another GP deliver care to the residents.

Another former care worker tells how Gordon, Lorraine and Nigel were trying to force a female resident to have her hair cut. As they tried to push her legs through the arms of a chair, the woman became increasingly 'panicky'. Gordon called the GP. Somehow, during the ensuing struggle, the woman wriggled free, losing her clothes in the process. Gordon, Lorraine and Nigel caught her, and held her down on the floor in the corner of the reception area.

By the time the GP arrived to deliver a sedative injection, the woman was still naked and lying pinned to the floor in the middle of the reception area. He apparently made no attempt to communicate with her or calm her down. 'There was no verbal,' she says. 'I was completely disgusted. She was on the floor in between the ladies' lounge and the stairs so everyone could see her.'

On another occasion, the same member of staff witnessed the GP giving flu jabs to the residents. 'They lined up and he gave them the jab. He didn't speak to them,' she says.

The relatives of the residents at Longcare raised concerns of a different nature about the medical care at the homes. After the Buckinghamshire inspection report was leaked, many of them were worried about the poor record-keeping and high prescription of sedatives, contraceptive injections and other drugs at Longcare.

They also wondered whether a GP who visited the homes so regularly and had an overview of the health and welfare of all the residents could or should have acted on that knowledge. They point in particular to the bruises, lack of cleanliness, ulcers, gum disorders, the rapid weight loss of new residents, the anal bleeding of the men and the vaginal infections of the women (a list of symptoms collated by June Raybaud, a former barrister and aunt of Janet Ward, during the court case and the many meetings of the families of the victims).

It is not at all clear how the medication regime was organised at the homes, but Rowe would of course have tried to hide as much as he could from outsiders. Rowe had learned how to be careful with signs of physical abuse during his Broadmoor days. He was a well-respected figure and it is possible that he simply blamed other residents for any bruises or signs that might indicate sexual trauma.

Janet
One day in 1994, out of the blue and before they learned of the inspection unit's investigation, a care worker rang Pauline Hennessey and told her Janet had started to become 'disruptive' and 'aggressive'. She was having outbursts almost every week. Previously, they would happen once a year, if at all.

Pauline drove down to Stoke Place for a meeting with her father, Janet's social worker, Nigel Rowe, Ray Cradock and the GP. They told her Janet would often enter a room and just start throwing furniture around. On one occasion, she grabbed a knife from the kitchen and threatened to kill herself.

'I told them I didn't understand what was going on because we had never had these problems before,' says Pauline. Despite being professionals in the field, 'They all looked at each other and said: "We have no idea either."'

When someone suggested that Janet could be placed in a secure unit, Pauline was horrified. Nothing was decided, but within a month, Cradock and Rowe told Pauline that Janet would have to find a new home.

It was only a few weeks later that Pauline was told by Janet's social worker about Buckinghamshire's investigation. She couldn't understand why the allegations hadn't been mentioned at the meeting at Stoke Place. When she phoned Longcare, Cradock told her they couldn't say anything because it was 'sub-judice'.

'I saw Janet falling apart and there was nothing I could do to help. Dr —'s first allegiance is to Janet,' she says. 'I can remember him being so patronising and the pure lack of help. I saw Janet falling apart and there was nothing I could do to help.'

Pauline was also mystified as to why the allegations hadn't been mentioned at the meeting at Longcare, just a few weeks earlier. 'They all knew Gordon Rowe had been banned from the premises, that he was accused of sexual abuse and that Janet was one of the "favourites", but they all sat there and said they didn't know what the problem was. I saw Janet falling apart and there was nothing I could do to help her.'

Linda

Rose Terry, whose sister Linda was a Longcare resident, remembers her becoming 'very quiet' while she was a resident at Stoke Place. Rose believes this was because of the drugs she was being given.

After Linda left Longcare, her new carers and new GP began to reduce the levels of sedatives. She is now on a much lower dose. 'She leads as normal life as she can. She is a completely different person now, compared to what she was before,' says Rose.

Stefano

After Desmond Tully left Longcare in 1990, Gordon Rowe became more prominent in Stefano Tunstell's care. Stefano's parents became increasingly concerned at how many drugs he was being fed, his weight loss, behavioural problems and incontinence.

Lidia, Stefano's mother, says Rowe was 'quite rude' in the spring of

1992 when they questioned the quantity of drugs her son was being given. At first, the drugs made him sleepy. Then the drugs were changed and he would become incredibly agitated. His parents' concerns increased when he returned home for a weekend visit, as he did every four or five weeks.

When he first moved to Stoke Place, Stefano had come home clean and shaved, but on this particular weekend they were shocked by the change in their son. The slight, curly haired young man was dressed in dirty, torn clothes. He was unshaven and appeared drawn and tense. He weighed just six and a half stone. He had always been slim, but his weight had never before dropped below seven stone. Stefano spent hours pacing backwards and forwards around the house or just sitting in a chair, avoiding the hugs of his parents, rocking backwards and forwards, playing with a piece of paper. Before Stoke Place, he had had good table manners. 'He started to eat in a way which was terrible,' says Lidia. 'It was like an animal, it was so fast, and he was getting so thin.'

Before he moved to Longcare, Stefano had been on 1.5mg of Haloperidol, a tranquiliser. By 1992, after he had moved to Longcare, the dose had increased to 20mg, four times a day. 'That was when we started to see he was very heavily drugged,' says Lidia.

In the following weeks, Lidia and Leslie became even more concerned. They had already noticed Stefano's incontinence, which had developed only since he moved to Stoke Place. They had contacted Surrey social services at the beginning of the summer, but were told not to worry. Now Stefano returned home for another weekend visit, and his mother was appalled to notice he was bleeding from the anus.

She told Stefano's social worker and a meeting was finally set up at the end of October with Longcare staff. Ray Cradock was there, as was the GP. The Tunstells were presented with a 'dreadful' report, written by Gordon Rowe. It described Stefano's inappropriate sexual behaviour around the house and in front of female residents, his habit of excitedly running into toilets and then running straight out again, and smearing himself with his own faeces.

Rowe's report also complained that Mr and Mrs Tunstell were undermining Stefano's care by questioning the amount of drugs he was being given. He even threatened to take them to court. The couple were 'horrified' that their sensitive son was suddenly being labelled a 'sex maniac'. This was not the son the Tunstells remembered, and there was no satisfactory explanation of the bleeding.

Lidia says they questioned the GP about the high levels of drugs he was prescribing Stefano. He 'said he could give Stefano as many drugs as he wanted and he said he wasn't even giving him as many as he thought he really needed. He was really horrible.'

Stefano was removed from Longcare in January, 1993. After a short spell back at home, Stefano started five months at an assessment unit, where medical staff began to lower his medication. The staff there confirmed to Lidia that the doses Stefano was being given were indeed too high.

He was also inspected by a police surgeon and a community nurse, who told the family his anus was 'full of scars'. But by this time, it was too long since the alleged abuse had occurred to draw any firm conclusions.

The Tunstells have since been told that Stefano may have suffered permanent kidney damage. They fear that it was a result of years of over-medication

(An unnamed resident)
Stefano does not seem to have been the only resident who was found to have been suffering from anal bleeding. Months before the Tunstells had met with the GP at Longcare, another resident had shown similar symptoms. According to Buckinghamshire's inspection unit report, the male resident had been taken to see a doctor after several days of severe bleeding.

The Independent Longcare Inquiry focused on the role of the county council and so its terms of reference did not include the medical care provided at the homes. Nonetheless, Tom Burgner, who led the inquiry, told me in an interview that he had been worried about treatment the residents received at the home. In the annexe of his official inquiry report, he specifically included the concerns of Stefano's parents (without mentioning the GP by name). The annexe also states that a woman from family 1 'was given a contraceptive by injection without her guardians consent', and that family 3 also had concerns about medication and how, once it was monitored away from Stoke Place by a consultant, the medication was 'reduced substantially'.

Dr Philippa Russell, a colleague of Burgner on the inquiry, remembers specific evidence presented concerning the GP. 'His collusion with the privacy, or the isolation, of the houses was, I think, very significant,' she told me. She highlighted his habit of visiting the residents at Stoke Place, rather than asking them to attend his surgery. This increased the isolation of the home and made it much less likely that another health professional-such as a practice nurse or dietician- would spot a problem.'

'There were a lot of criticisms of him among the local doctors... They were worried about how he always went to Longcare. He saw the residents personally, individually, when he visited the home, in a way that other people wouldn't. I think it was inconceivable that he would not have had his suspicions. He may have had difficulty getting evidence, but he must have had some idea of what was going on.'

Over the years, I made repeated calls to the General Medical Council's press office about the GP, in relation to the complaints I had heard about the care he provided at Longcare. Usually, there was no comment. The GMC's line on such cases is always to make no comment unless and until it decides to proceed with a public inquiry by its professional conduct committee. The GP also declined to comment when I approached him on at least three occasions.

So it was not until October 2003 that I discovered by chance that the GMC had been approached in 1996 by Thames Valley Police with concerns about the possibility of 'substandard record-keeping and irresponsible prescribing' by the GP. It seems they felt they lacked the expertise to assess this issue and wanted to pass it on to the relevant professional body. The GMC had considered this information, but 'decided that the allegations didn't raise an issue of serious professional misconduct' on the part of the GP. The case was closed with no further investigation by the GMC.

These concerns of Thames Valley Police were not mentioned when, in November 1996, Gary Deacon's parents also filed a complaint with the GMC. They were concerned at how the GP had handled Gary's care between 1990 and 1996. Throughout that time, there had been just two brief entries in his medical records. They were also angry that, in 1996, the doctor's medical practice had taken five months to act on a report from an epilepsy specialist prescribing medication for partial seizures.

Staff at Longcare had responded to Gary's behavioural problems the only way they knew how—by drugging him with sedatives, the sedatives that had been prescribed by the GP. His parents were shocked to arrive one afternoon and find Gary hardly conscious and 'zombyish'. They switched to a new GP, who reduced the medication, and Gary's condition gradually improved.

The GMC told the Deacons in June 1997 that the GP had been 'dismayed' to learn of the 'administrative oversight' which led to the letter from the consultant being filed without any action. The GP 'outlined the steps which have been taken at the surgery to improve their administrative procedures, and is confident that such oversights will not be repeated,' they were told.

In the case of a patient with epilepsy and a learning disability, such as Gary, one imagines accurate notes are kept. The GP told the GMC that he 'made appropriate entries for the infrequent occasions that Gary required medical attention'. The Deacons disagreed. The GMC replied to the Deacons: 'Clearly, although I noted your comments in our telephone conversation of 23 April that he would have certainly had "treatment" more than twice in a five year period, the GMC is not in a position to comment on whether Gary's treatment over this period only necessitated two entries.'

The GMC reiterated its 'guidance on the importance of keeping accurate patient records' to the GP, 'with a view to his future practice'. But it took no action to investigate the matter further.

June Raybaud, Janet Ward's aunt, however, was determined to force the medical authorities to carry out a more thorough investigation into the medical attention given at the homes. Raybaud, a barrister, contacted the GMC in 2000, two years after the Longcare inquiry had reported its findings, to ask the organisation to examine the GP's treatment of the Longcare residents. The GMC told her it had not seen the public inquiry report, published in 1998. She immediately sent a copy.

By January 2001, the GMC was liaising with Nicola Harney, Janet Ward's lawyer, over Raybaud's complaint. They told Harney in a letter that, because of their earlier 'investigation', they could not look at allegations of poor record-keeping and irresponsible prescribing again 'unless we receive significant new evidence to support the allegation'.

But it continued: 'If there was sexual or physical abuse and neglect and ill-treatment of the residents and, as Mrs Raybaud alleges, the principal medical carer... failed to act, then this would in principle seem like a new allegation as compared with those which concentrated on substandard record-keeping and irresponsible prescribing. There must be a duty for a doctor to report mistreatment of residents in a nursing home.'

By now, representatives of one of the victims had obtained legal aid to sue the GP for negligence. Harney commissioned a medical expert to write a report about the GP's treatment of a former Longcare resident, Michael S. The GMC asked to see this report when it was ready.

In December 2001, Harney sent a mass of documents to the GMC, including police statements from the trial, the inspection unit report, the expert report, and copies of Michael S's medical records. She also told the GMC that it could see all her other clients' medical records. Raybaud says this offer was never taken up by the GMC.

In April, 2002, the GMC requested Raybaud to make a 'statutory' declaration about her complaint and comment on all the witness statements Harney had sent to the GMC. Raybaud was flummoxed. She had already lodged her complaint and detailed her concerns about the GP. She was now being asked to comment on scores of witness statements compiled for the case against Buckinghamshire County Council; statements she had never seen and had no right to see.

Two months later, the GMC wrote to Raybaud saying that it was temporarily suspending its investigation, because of her failure to make this 'statutory declaration'.

In March 2003, three years after contacting the GMC, Raybaud received another letter. It confirmed that the GMC's Preliminary Proceedings Committee was again considering her allegations that the GP had failed to act over the ill-treatment of the Longcare residents.

The committee had read the expert's report. The letter noted that 'the lack of medical records was his most stringent criticism of Dr — but that he also had concerns with regard to prescribing and had concluded that Dr —'s practice was probably below what would be expected of a general practitioner'.

The GMC then told Raybaud that it was 'concerned' at this evidence of high levels of prescribing and the 'issues around the medical records' but 'noted that these had not been included in the allegations'.

In its response, the GMC seemed to have overlooked the fact that its own organisation had told Nicola Harney in January 2001 that it would be unable to consider allegations of record-keeping and irresponsible prescribing due to its earlier investigation. It was not June Raybaud who had failed to include the allegations in her complaint, but the GMC that had removed them from consideration.

The letter concluded by saying that the committee had adjourned the case against the GP to decide whether it could, after all, consider these issues.

Four months later, the GMC wrote to Raybaud again. The letter said that the expert's report on Michael S had criticised the GP's 'prescribing of lithium for Mr S and his failure to adequately monitor his blood whilst on this medication [and] also raised general concerns about the lack of records and the standard of those which had been kept, and the way in which sedative drugs were prescribed for the residents, to be administered by the carers.'

It claimed that, although the GP was the principal doctor treating the Longcare residents from 1990 to 1994, he was not the only GP to do so. It also stated that, when the GP visited Longcare on his weekly visits, he had seen residents in the reception area. (On the question whether this was or was not an appropriate place for a GP to conduct his surgery, the letter is silent.)

'The Committee considered that in such circumstances he was probably given very little opportunity to see what was happening in the home and could not necessarily be criticised for having failed to pick up any signs of abuse. The Committee felt that the perpetrators of the abuse no doubt took steps to ensure that it was not revealed to visitors to the home. Furthermore, the Committee considered that given Dr —'s role, he would probably have been limited as to where he could go and whom he could see in the home.'

These comments, perhaps more than any made by the GMC, seem to be suggestive of the way it conducted its 'investigation'. Instead of putting the question to the GP whether he had been limited to where he could go, it seems to have been satisfied to construe a self-made argument that he probably was. One strongly wonders whether the GMC asked the GP outright whether he had had any suspicions about the abuse and, if so, whether he had raised them with Longcare. And if he had, for what reasons he decided not to take his concerns elsewhere.

The letter then went on to state that the GP's representatives had pointed out to the committee that 'the Inquiry Report details how other organisations failed to discover any evidence of neglect or ill treatment even when they were specifically conducting investigations with these points in mind'.

Again the point this proves to the GMC is highly ambiguous. No organisation was in direct contact with the victims of the abuse the way the GP was. In the period leading up to the launch of the full scale investigation in November 1993, there was little if any contact between Bucks inspection officers and Longcare residents, except for the officer who interviewed Dorothy Abbott in April 1991 after her complaint about Gordon Rowe's violence assault. Unless the GMC's is suggesting other people's failures absolve GPs, the comment seems hardly relevant to the question of whether—from his own vantage point—the GP failed to pick up signs of abuse based on his privileged access to the victims and their health records.

The committee decided, in the light of legal advice, not to allow the addition of the 'extra' allegations concerning record-keeping and irresponsible prescribing. The letter concluded: 'It further determined that in the light of the inquiry report and the police investigations, there was insufficient evidence and no real prospect of further, sufficient evidence emerging in support of the allegations for serious professional misconduct to be established in this case.'

It also claimed that there had been no criticism of the GP 'by the Police or the Independent Inquiry'. This came as another surprise as it was the GMC which had informed Nicola Harney that Thames Valley Police had approached it in 1996 with concerns about 'possible substandard record-keeping and irresponsible prescribing' by the GP. In addition, the annexe of Burgner's independent inquiry report specified three cases of concern.

Apart from contacting the GP's representatives, it seems that the GMC launched no investigations of its own. It did not even contact the members of the Independent Longcare Inquiry to ensure that it was not overlooking evidence. For the third time the GMC failed to investigate whether the medical care offered at Longcare was acceptable, particularly in the light of the horrific abuse at the two homes. Where others, such as MPs, the government, and members of Thames Valley Police, had reacted to the revelation of the abuse in 1994 in a vigorous and responsible way, it is clear that the GMC has failed in its role as authoritative recourse for complaints and as the guardian of standards of medical practice.

June Raybaud is upset at what she sees as the GMC's failure to launch a proper investigation into the medical care provided to the residents of Longcare by the GP. 'The GMC behaved in a most mysterious and confused manner... They are not protecting anybody.' She believes the only option now left open to her is to call for a judicial review of the GMC's decision not to hold a full and proper inquiry into the case.

The GMC did pass its decision to the GP's local Primary Care Trust. Its chief executive, Mike Attwood, told me the GP's case raised serious issues about the way people with learning difficulties are treated by general practitioners. He calls for updated guidance for GPs on how to treat people with learning difficulties and for this to be given national service framework status. This would impose a formal obligation on all GPs to follow the guidelines.

He also calls for formal mechanisms to force different regulators to work together on inspections of health and care facilities. 'There ought to be a formal duty of partnership,' he said. 'What the problem seems to be is that there is no statutory obligation for that to happen.'

He was also concerned at how long the GMC took to deal with the complaint. 'As a new chief executive in a new organisation which didn't exist (at the time), one has to ask why it all took such a long time.'

Curiously, the GMC did not make Mike Attwood aware of its previous two investigations. He has said that he will now look at them as well.

Meanwhile, because of its refusal to answer questions about its deliberations, a catalogue of vital questions remain about the way the General Medical Council dealt with the complaints against the GP.

Why did the GMC not interview the members of the Independent Longcare Inquiry, Tom Burgner and Philippa Russell? Why did it apparently fail to take up Nicola Harney's offer to forward copies of the medical records of her clients? Why did it speak only with representatives of the GP in question? Why did the GMC state in its July 2003 letter to June Raybaud that the police had made no criticism of the GP, when Thames Valley Police had approached it in 1996? Why did it not launch a full and proper investigation of its own at that time? Or when the Deacons lodged their complaint? Or when Raybaud lodged hers?

The final question the GMC's conduct raises is whether this is the way it would have dealt with a complaint made about a GP's treatment of patients without learning difficulties? Has its failure to investigate the GP's conduct been merely a repetition of the many failures of Buckinghamshire County Council to exercise its powers properly?

One wonders whether this just another example of the GMC's inability to investigate Britain's doctors. A notorious recent case, where the main perpetrator was himself a doctor, illustrates the GMC's inability to regulate its profession. Dr Harold Shipman killed his first patient, Eva Lyons, in March 1975. He was convicted in February 1976 of obtaining pethidine by forgery and deception to feed his addiction to the drug. Later that year he obtained enough morphine to kill 360 people, supposedly for one patient. Even after receiving psychiatric and drug treatment, Shipman was allowed to return to work as a GP. Even when he was fired from the Todmorden medical practice for forging prescriptions, he received a heavy fine but was not struck off by the

GMC, but simply sent a warning letter. Even after his arrest in February 1999, the GMC failed to strike him off the register for another year. Had the GMC investigated sooner, some of the 215 murdered patients might have been saved.

The case of Harold Shipman is very different from the involvement of the medical profession at Longcare. At the heart of Longcare stands Gordon Rowe. Yet, crucially, Rowe's cynical regime prospered through overmedication and could not have succeeded without it. Until regulatory bodies such as the GMC ensure that they conduct full and proper investigations when questions are raised about those they are meant to regulate, public confidence and safety will remain greatly diminished.

30. The Legal System

> 'The Crown Prosecution Service do not want to know. They put it in the 'too difficult' box. Why don't they have some experts to deal with these cases? You can have as many laws as you like, but if the CPS aren't prepared to put the work in to prosecute these cases, you might as well forget it.'
>
> Mother of autistic teenager sexually assaulted by convicted paedophile;
> January, 2001

If Gordon Rowe's family and friends were devastated by his suicide, so were the police officers who had spent eighteen months piecing together a case against him. They had already struggled to overcome the initial double foul-up perpetrated by their own force. With Rowe's death, 90 per cent of this work was rendered useless.

They now had to pick up the pieces of the investigation and consider whether there was anyone else they should prosecute. Bound met the Crown's QC, Jonathan Caplan, and his assistant, Amanda Pinto. They decided to prosecute Angela Rowe, Desmond Tully and Lorraine Field, and also consider prosecuting Longcare.

Bound was disappointed when the Director of Public Prosecutions ruled out a prosecution of Rowe's company. 'We wanted to prove that out of the misery inflicted on seventy residents, Gordon Rowe had made a lot of money. We thought that if we were to prosecute the company and fail, we could push for a change in the law,' he said.

A Crown Prosecution Service spokeswoman told me there was no law that could have been used to prosecute Longcare. 'Criminal law is all about individuals, not companies, apart from some very specific areas,' she said. So Rowe's company, which made huge profits for its shareholders from the abusive regime, escaped criminal sanction.

The trial of Angela Rowe, Lorraine Field and Desmond Tully at Kingston Crown Court—which began on April 14, 1997—was not going to reflect the true gravity of what had happened. Because of Gordon Rowe's suicide, the jury would hear nothing of the sexual assaults, rapes and the most brutal aspects of the Longcare regime. His death also meant that none of the residents would be called to give evidence. Although it undoubtedly saved some of his victims a measure of distress, it also deprived them of the right to have their day in court, to have their voices heard.

The trial lasted just under four weeks. Without testimony from former residents, the jury relied mostly on prosecution evidence from ex-members of staff and expert witnesses.

There was little evidence submitted by the defence. Apart from the defendants' pleas of innocence, there were only a few character witnesses who praised Desmond Tully's residential home in Devon, and a couple of healthcare specialists who testified to Longcare's fine qualities. None of Gordon's former police friends found the time to make it to Kingston, although it had been rumoured that one police officer might give evidence on behalf of Angela Rowe.

In the end, after several days of jury deliberation, Angela Rowe was found guilty of two counts of ill-treatment and two of neglect. Although the police had also charged her with indecently assaulting a male resident, Gary Deacon, the prosecution had decided not to complicate the case, and asked for the charge to remain on the court's files. None of the evidence concerning the allegation was heard during the trial.

Rowe had described herself in court as nothing more than 'a glorified housekeeper', but the jury didn't believe her. They heard how she had ordered Jackie, a middle-aged woman with Down's syndrome, to eat meals outside as a punishment; pulled another woman with Down's syndrome down a flight of stairs by her hair; and 'wilfully neglected' two residents by depriving them of toiletries to save money.

Angela Rowe cut a sorry figure. She was taking Prozac for depression and other drugs to combat anorexia. Halfway through the trial, she received a warning from the judge after allegedly confronting a witness outside the court and threatening to 'fucking kill' her for 'lying'.

Lorraine Field was found guilty of three counts of ill-treatment. The court was told how Field screamed abuse at residents, hit those who annoyed her and took part in the punishment meted out to Jackie. A fourth charge, an allegation that she had sat on Janet Ward and poured jugs of cold water over her head to 'calm her down' was left on the files after the jury failed to reach a verdict.

Tully was convicted of a single count of ill-treatment. The jury had listened as a former member of staff described how he forcefully administered an enema to a middle-aged woman and slapped her on her bare buttock when she tried to struggle. He was cleared of punching two other residents, with a fourth charge left on the files.

Four other charges—two against Rowe and one each against Tully and Field—had been dismissed earlier in the case on the orders of the judge, because of a lack of evidence.

Monday, May 12, 1997. Court Six, Kingston Crown Court
Angela Rowe's eyes appeared glazed as she walked between the young man—a friend of the Rowe family who had supported her throughout the trial—and her solicitor towards the court exit. To her right, several of the victims' relatives in the public gallery were on their feet, staring at her, but she didn't notice them either. She walked past the small group of reporters and court officials and walked through the light wood double-doors.

When Duncan Thomson, Angela Rowe's solicitor, visited her at home later that day, he found her still in a condition of deep shock. Her barrister, Stephen Kramer QC, later told the court she was 'alternately gibbering as if she was a little girl', asking for her husband, and telling those around her she 'didn't like the sound of doors slamming'. Whether this was all a show in a last-ditch attempt to wring sympathy from the judge is unclear.

Four weeks later, Angela Rowe was jailed for two-and-a-half years, despite Kramer telling the judge his client would 'rather die' than suffer the shame of a prison sentence. Field, too, was jailed—for fifteen months. Tully received a fine.

Among the relatives of the victims, there were some expressions of satisfaction or relief, but none of triumph. Several of them, including Janet Ward's sister, Pauline, had attended much of the trial and heard for themselves the evidence of former members of staff. It had been a deeply distressing experience, particularly so for Pauline, because the jury had been unable to reach a verdict on a charge that Lorraine Field had ill-treated Janet.

Barbara McCarthy, whose son Shaun was abused at the homes, and was at the court throughout the trial with her husband, Terry, said after the sentencing: 'I'm glad they got sent down. They deserved it, regardless of how long it is. Now they might know what it is like to be locked away for hours and days on end, like some of the residents were.'

June Raybaud added: 'I think the judge took into account the seriousness of the offences and the fact that these people were so vulnerable.'

Jon Bound, the Supt on the case, also welcomed the sentences and paid tribute to the police officers whose painstaking work led to the convictions. He mentioned by name the trio who had been at court during the trial, acting as assistants for the barristers, and soothing the nerves of prosecution witnesses—Madeleine Stewart, Cathy Woodliffe and Denise Jenkins. It was, he said, 'one of the most complex investigations undertaken by Thames Valley Police, but was necessary to protect some of the most vulnerable members of our community'.

As the trial ended, Judge Baker demanded a change in the law. He said the powers of the Mental Health Act had provided him with inadequate sentencing powers and there was an urgent need for a parliamentary review of the relevant laws. The press called for an inquiry into the role of Buckinghamshire County Council in the outrage, which took place several months later.

Bound also called for new legislation, with tighter inspection and registration guidelines. 'Those involved,' he said, 'should not be allowed to make vast profits at the expense of other people's misery.'

Perhaps most markedly, he warned: 'If these matters are happening in Slough, then they are occurring elsewhere in the country, and we have already been contacted by other forces involved in similar investigations.'

31. The Other Local Authorities

'Two teenagers who kicked to death a man who went to the aid of his mentally handicapped son as they tried to bully him were jailed yesterday. Ray Steadman, 18, and Christopher Bryan, 17, both from Dagenham, east London, must serve 10 years before parole is considered.'

The Independent, June 9, 2001

As my research into Longcare reached its end, proof began to emerge of yet another serious failure in the system; one that dated all the way back to the introduction of institutional care for the 'mentally defective' in the middle of the nineteenth century.

Gordon Rowe knew when he set up Longcare in 1983 that there was a severe shortage of residential homes for learning disabled people. Thousands of patients were being resettled into the community from the long-stay hospitals. Many of these people had been living in such institutions since they were very young children, often for more than 50 years. This was exaggerating the tensions in the residential care system, and people like Rowe, with his social work contacts, were well placed to take advantage.

The district health authorities, which ran the hospitals, were faced with a drastic shortage of potential placements. They were also acting under the authority of inadequate legislation that was open to widely differing interpretations.

Once a patient was found a home in the community and had spent six months settling in, he or she was 'discharged' by the hospital. Money to pay for their care was passed by the Department of Health and Social Security to the patient's regional health authority, which usually delegated it to its relevant district health authority. This district health authority could then reach an agreement to transfer the funding to its social services department. But local and health authorities often failed to reach such agreements. Responsibility frequently remained instead with the health authority.

A further complication was that it was not always clear to which area a former patient 'belonged'. If they had been at the hospital since before 1970, they would become the responsibility of that hospital's regional health authority. But if they had arrived at the hospital more recently than 1970, their own 'home' regional health authority would become responsible for finding them somewhere to live.

Confused? So, it seems, were the authorities. One senior social care figure, Anne*, laid much of the blame at the feet of the Department of Health. 'The department used to talk about collaboration. The theory was that, if you were in a hospital and you needed to be placed outside, as people with learning disabilities did, there should have been a co-ordinated approach and a suitable placement for you should be found and ongoing support. It didn't work like that,' she told me. 'There is a can of worms waiting to be opened up.'

Dr Jean Collins, director of Values Into Action, which promotes the rights of people with learning difficulties, told me: 'The government had no grip at all. They didn't do anything about it. They just let it go on. The Government had no idea about what was going on on the ground.'

Dr Collins, who described the chaos caused by the resettlement process in her book, *The Resettlement Game*, believes the health authorities that retained responsibility for their former patients during the 80s simply dropped them in their new placements and forgot about them. 'In many cases they just didn't check up. They would just get a recurring bill and pay it. Residential care for people with learning disabilities is incredibly expensive, but they didn't check up to see what they were getting.'

A Department of Health spokeswoman made it clear that the responsibility for ensuring appropriate arrangements were in place lay with the health authorities. There had been confusion in some cases where placements had broken down as to who was responsible, she admitted, and the department had issued 'clarifying' guidance in 1992. As for whether the department itself was partly responsible for this mistake, she declined to comment.

Nobody seemed to know who was supposed to be looking out for these people. And, if they did know, they didn't seem particularly bothered about it. The former patients were often left at the mercy of the people who ran their new homes, without a social worker or nurse to keep a regular check on their welfare.

The seventeen former Botley's Park patients moved to Stoke Place during late 1983 and 1984 and were some of Longcare's first residents. Among them were Dorothy Abbott and her boyfriend, Jimmy.

Dorothy moved to Stoke Place in December, 1983. She was officially discharged from Botley's six months later. Then for the next five years, nothing.

Dorothy entered a kind of social care No-Man's Land. South-West Thames Regional Health Authority—which covered Botley's Park—was still responsible for her welfare. It continued to pay the bills for her care, but, once she was discharged, none of its officers or nurses visited her to check on her welfare. She was finally 'picked up' by the Royal London

Borough of Kingston-upon-Thames in 1989, but only after her sister contacted its social services department to express concern about Stoke Place.

Jenny Webb, head of community care services for Kingston, was unable to work out who had been responsible for Dorothy before Kingston took over her case. 'I don't think it is terribly clear,' she told me. 'I am not clear that anyone took any overview responsibility. Certainly we were not notified of the placement. Obviously, in terms of the standards you would expect with any placement of a vulnerable person, it is a matter of concern.'

Further evidence came from the London Borough of Merton. Two Botley's patients, Edwin and Derek, were placed at Longcare in 1983; again, it seems, by South-West Thames Regional Health Authority. In April 1986, the two men became Merton's responsibility, when the council was asked to provide 'top-up' funding for them, following changes to benefits legislation. In those three years, they hadn't been visited once by a health or social worker.

Merton council's policy was to only review out-of-borough clients every two years, due to 'demand and limited resources', so Edwin and Derek were not reviewed for the first time by a social worker until 1988, five years after moving to Longcare.

Another example of this chaotic approach comes from the London Borough of Richmond. Three former long-stay hospital patients who originated from Richmond were placed at Longcare.

It took the council more than a year to come up with the following answer to my question: how frequently did you visit your clients while they were at the homes?

'Having searched through all the relevant files, the available evidence suggests that people with learning disabilities who were placed at Stoke Place and originated from the London Borough of Richmond upon Thames were visited on average at regular intervals during the period for which the borough had financial responsibility.'

'On average at regular intervals'. Only a local authority could come up with such a meaningless phrase. When pressed, the reason became apparent.

Stewart Ruston, community services manager for Kingston and Richmond Joint Service for People with Learning Disabilities, told me that at some stage the responsibility for the trio had passed from the health authority (South-West Thames again) to the council. But exactly when it passed, he didn't know. 'I cannot find anything that specifies what, when, where, how,' he admitted.

There are no records of any visits to the trio until the early 90s. And during the 80s? 'Obviously, there were some visits, but I do not know if there is a lack of information. We probably didn't accept responsibility until they had been there for quite some period. A year or so or more. It's not clear for all three of them.'

'The recording practices were not as good as they are now. I don't know if things were done and not recorded... or not done. From our records, we can't prove either way. There were gaps. You can assume neglect, or assume that things would have been done but were not recorded because of poor practice.'

This conclusion was the result of scores of letters and telephone calls from me over fifteen months. To sum up: a scandalous lack of proper records, no clear idea of whether Richmond's social workers did their job properly, and not the least idea of when the responsibility passed from health authority to council.

But it was not only former patients of the long-stay hospitals who had been abandoned at Longcare, as the detectives investigating the allegations against Gordon Rowe in the autumn of 1994 had discovered.

The majority of the homes' residents had been placed there by local councils. Madeleine Stewart, one of the officers who worked on the 18-month investigation, told me: 'It soon became clear to us that many of the 26 local authorities with clients at Longcare had had little or no contact with them for years. Some were not even aware they had residents at the homes.'

Most were placed there by London boroughs, many of which were desperately short of residential homes within their own areas. Often, the only option was to find places outside London. Stoke Place, and later Stoke Green, both less than 20 miles from the western edge of the capital, were perfectly situated to mop up some of this excess demand.

Gus Gray, who turned down an application by Rowe to open a large residential home in Berkshire in 1985, believes the Longcare boss knew that social workers from local authorities outside Bucks would 'fall over themselves' to place clients at Stoke Place. 'Stoke Place seldom had any vacancies, although Rowe was quite often prepared to squeeze people in, and that is always a dangerous sign. It means that somebody else is being squeezed.'

'The reason inappropriate placements are made is that in terms of residential accommodation, there is no slack in the system,' he said. 'Residential care is more expensive than living at home and the social services budget is constrained. Because long-term planning is difficult, they are forced from time to time to have to find a long-term bed in a short space of time. That enables people like Rowe to say: "Well, yes, I have got a room in the dogs' kennels or the stables."'

Rowe also had a reputation for taking 'problem' clients rejected by other services. 'Many placing authorities which were forced to find places where problem clients could be accommodated, didn't inquire too deeply into what was going on,' Gray told me.

Unfortunately, the London boroughs were also short of funds. Social services budgets were squeezed in real terms throughout the 80s and 90s. They were also short of social workers. One former social worker said there were 'an awful lot of problems and nobody was addressing them.'

'If you have a series of crises on your desk, people in residential care tend to have less attention. That's the kind of pressure that exists for most social workers. We have a duty to the well-being of everybody... but if there are people in acute need, they inevitably get the first bite of the cherry. It depends on whether you have enough social workers to keep the pressures at an acceptable level. I am bound to say there are not enough resources and there are not enough social workers.

'There were a lot of mentally handicapped people. London boroughs used to farm them out and there was no follow up. You couldn't possibly do anything more, because your caseload was too high. It was in the "Planned Neglect" pile, because you knew you ought to do something about it, but it got shoved down to the bottom of the pile.'

Inevitably, those who are seen as being in 'acute need' are those whose problems have been spotted by social services. Those who cannot speak up for themselves are often assumed to be OK, so they find themselves at the bottom of the pile. Once you're at the bottom of the pile, it's almost impossible to find a way out.

Ian Johnston, director of the British Association of Social Workers, told me: 'One of the features is that you have to be a problem before you see a social worker. It's a resource question. There are a lot of well-intentioned people in social work, they want to do a good job, but they are simply stretched too far and the expectations placed on them are unrealistic.'

As for the Longcare residents? 'They were out of sight, out of mind.'

One care assistant, who worked at Stoke Place for five years, told me: 'We never saw any social workers for the residents. If the social workers had bothered to come to us, I think we would have told them. I don't think half of them had social workers.'

Shaun McCarthy, who is autistic and has a learning difficulty, was moved to Stoke Place in September, 1987, by the London Borough of Waltham Forest. Shaun's social worker visited Stoke Place in December, 1987, and again, six months later. He visited him once more in March, 1989. After that, Shaun wasn't seen by his social worker for more than 18 months.

Ron Wallace, Waltham Forest's executive director of community services, told me that all these case reviews 'concluded that Shaun was appropriately placed'. But Shaun's parents, Barbara and Terry, remember being visited at their London home by his social worker every year. They say they were told that it was Buckinghamshire's job to inspect Stoke Place.

Following a review in November, 1990, Shaun's social worker didn't visit him again until September, 1994, after Bucks County Council had sent Waltham Forest a copy of its Longcare abuse report.

Shaun was fortunate that Barbara and Terry visited him every two or three weeks. They noticed the lack of staff, the occasional injuries to their son, how Shaun's new clothes would always be 'lost in the laundry', his weight loss and the high levels of medication. But they did not have the training or experience to conclude that Shaun was being abused. The person who might have been able to do that, had he visited Stoke Place regularly, was Shaun's social worker. But in four years Shaun did not receive a single visit from Waltham Forest social services.

Wallace told me: 'Clearly, I would have preferred that reviews had continued at regular intervals. I wish I could say that had reviews and visits continued, the pattern of abuse at Stoke Place would have come to light. Unfortunately, even with the most intensive visiting, abuse has frequently gone undetected.'

But the council had 'learned many lessons from this experience'. Waltham Forest now allocates social workers to all residents in long term care and seeks 'regular feedback' from relatives and inspectors. It is also trying to place as many learning disabled people as possible in homes within the borough.

Unfortunately, Shaun's is far from being the most worrying case. The London Borough of Tower Hamlets was asked during the Buckinghamshire inspection unit investigation whether it had any clients at Longcare. No, said the council's social services department.

When this response was queried, Tower Hamlets' director of social services ordered a search of council records and discovered that there *was* a Tower Hamlets client living at Longcare. Rosie Valton had been living at Stoke Place since January, 1984. She had been repeatedly raped and beaten by Gordon Rowe.

Tower Hamlets declined to discuss the case with me, or to detail the number of visits Rosie received from a social worker at Stoke Place.

One social services consultant says Rosie's case is 'a significant example of the lack of safeguards' that exists. He believes much of social work today is spent in 'crisis intervention work'. 'There are many people that are placed somewhere and their cases are closed or they don't have an allocated care manager [social worker]. That is happening in an increasing number of cases. It is one way of cutting down the workload.'

But it was not just the London boroughs that were failing their clients. In fact, Berkshire was itself forced to place Gary Deacon with Rowe at Stoke Place—against Gus Gray's wishes—because it could find nowhere else for him to live.

Stefano Tunstell was placed at Stoke Place late in 1987. He was visited three times in 1988, as his social worker from Surrey County Council oversaw efforts to settle him into his new home. But he wasn't visited again until February, 1991. In the summer of 1992, his parents began to raise serious concerns about the standard of care he was receiving. He was finally visited once more in October, 1992.

Georgie Agass, spokeswoman for Surrey County Council, told me: 'It's not usual for a person who is in a placement outside of the county to be visited more than once a year.' This is the frightening irony of the situation: it is often those who are placed a long distance away from their friends and family who are most at risk. But it is these clients who are visited least often, because it is too expensive for the placing authorities to travel to see them.

Agass said Surrey was battling social services budget cuts throughout the 80s and 90s, as were other authorities. By 2000, each care manager had responsibility for close to 100 clients.

Nicky Power was another client failed by her local authority. She was one of the first Longcare residents, and lived there for nearly 10 years. She was visited by her social worker from Kent County Council in late 1983 and early 1984 (probably to make sure she was settled in) and then again later in 1984. There was a gap of more than two years until the next visit in

1987. She was visited twice in 1988, but at some stage during that year her social worker left the council for another job. She wasn't replaced.

Nicky was visited by somebody from social services in 1989 and 1991 for an annual review, but wasn't seen again until the Powers found out by accident three years later that she didn't have her own social worker. Throughout this period, Nicky was being raped by Gordon Rowe.

A spokeswoman for Kent social services said a 'team leader' would have been responsible for Nicky's case, but she would not have had a named social worker. Mr and Mrs Power say they didn't receive any information about Nicky from the council for nearly six years. 'After the social worker left I think she was probably at the bottom of the pile,' says Susan Power. 'We didn't have any contact for a long time. We didn't think there was anything to worry about, so we didn't complain.'

Some local authorities do seem to have made regular visits to the Longcare homes to check up on their clients and monitor their progress.

The London Borough of Harrow, for instance, placed two residents with Longcare. One, who was there for seven years, was visited nine times, in addition to numerous letters and telephone calls. The other was there for five years and was visited fourteen times. Again, there were many letters and telephone calls, and none of this produced any evidence of ill-treatment or assaults. This illustrates how difficult it can be for social workers to build up the kind of trusting relationship with a client that can lead to a disclosure of abuse, when they see them only once or maybe twice a year.

Hertfordshire County Council visited its male client at Longcare three or four times a year while he was at Stoke Place, and 'spent some time alone with him on each visit', and again found no cause for concern.

The London Borough of Havering visited its clients—including Janet Ward and Simon Scott—two or three times a year, as well as attending annual reviews. There were also frequent visits from Janet's and Simon's relatives.

The disturbing message is that, even with regular visits, there is no guarantee that social workers will realise that abuse is taking place. Rowe was practised at covering up all signs of abuse when he knew outsiders were around. And every time a social worker visited for an annual review, it was arranged in advance with Longcare. Rowe had plenty of notice of when social workers were going to be poking their noses into his affairs. It was easy for him to ensure that he, his staff and his residents were on their best behaviour.

In any case, for every local authority that did manage to send a social worker at least once a year to check up on their client, there were two or three that did not.

Tom Burgner was concerned about the lack of regular visits by social workers. 'Of course, we would have wanted the placing authorities to take a lot more interest in the people they had placed,' he said.

His fellow inquiry member, Dr Philippa Russell, told me that Jean Jeffrey, Buckinghamshire's director of social services, had written in December 1993 to every one of the local authorities with Longcare clients to warn them that they were investigating complaints about the home. 'There was absolutely not a flicker of interest,' said Dr Russell.

She experienced a similar situation in the mid-90s. 'It was a private children's home, which a lot of London authorities had put children in. A lot of concerns were being raised about what was going on at the home. The director of the host authority's social services department wrote to all the placement authorities and said he was very concerned about the home. He did not believe it was a safe place. They had not been able to get evidence which the local police thought would stand up in court, particularly because of the severity of the disability of the children. None of them could speak. He expressed the view really quite strongly and said if he had placed a child in such a home, he would have removed him. He didn't get a single reply and when he rang the various local authorities, they said, "well, we have nowhere else to put them." I think that illustrates the dilemma.'

She believes that the attitude of local authorities to the clients they place in out-of-area services is 'one of the most shocking things about the management of residential care'.

James Churchill, chief executive of the Association for Residential Care, whose members are responsible for about 14,000 residential places for learning disabled people, agrees. 'It's all a question of money and resources and time. Once the placement is made and the finances sorted out, our members' experience is that you are often left to get on with it.'

Fiona Mactaggart, Slough's MP, added: 'In effect what had happened was that a bunch of people had got lost, except to the finance department. They just featured as bills. I wonder sometimes how many people there are around Britain whose only contact with anyone who has any kind of responsibility for them is someone just paying a bill. Because I bet that wasn't unique and I bet it still happens.'

Six years after the Longcare case was exposed, a study published by the Norah Fry Research Centre[1] found that disabled children placed in residential schools were often not visited by social workers or education officers. One education officer told the researchers: 'Once the youngster is at the school, on a day to day basis it's the school's responsibility to ensure the welfare of the child, though we do get reports from the school via the annual review process.' If it is still this relaxed with children, it will be far worse with adults.

During my research, I had heard stories of coaches of patients being shipped up from London to residential homes in the north during the 80s, because of the drastic shortage of places in the capital. This would have placed these people even further from relatives and friends than the residents of Longcare. So, in the summer of 2003, I decided to try to find out whether what happened at Longcare was an isolated occurrence, or whether the practice of sending vulnerable adults to distant placements far from their original homes was still being repeated across the country.

It quickly became clear that many social care professionals shared my concerns. In Lincolnshire, for example, I was told there were 570 people living there who were originally from out of county. Many of those from the London boroughs, I was told by a senior manager, were believed to be not receiving annual visits from social workers. Many had been placed in homes where they are at serious risk of abuse.

In Kent, the problem was 'rife', said Simon Hewson, head of psychology for East Kent Mental Health and Social Care Partnership Trust. He said it was 'pretty rare' for such people to receive more than one visit a year from their social worker. Often, they did not even get that. 'People are just left,' he said. He believes there are hundreds of people in such situations in Kent. And, as in Lincolnshire, some of the homes they have been placed in are 'pretty shady'.

Dr Collins said she too believes, 'anecdotally', that many people in out of area placements are not being visited at all by social workers. 'Nobody has any records or statistics, but I think it is widespread. The reason I think it is widespread is that wherever I go in the country, people talk to me about it being a problem. They are concerned that people are being abandoned by their paying authority.'

I spoke to Steven Rose, chief executive of Choice Support, which provides supported living and residential care to people with learning difficulties. He agrees with Collins. 'In my experience,' he told me, 'local authorities' supervision and follow-up of placements after they have made them are absolutely abysmal.'

He estimates that every London borough has about 100 learning disabled clients in out-of-area placements.

'Even in their own borough, they rarely get round them once a year. I know they do not get to the ones that are miles away. They just haven't got the resources. It is a very real problem. We know that any vulnerable person is more likely to be financially, emotionally, physically or sexually abused. We know there is a high incidence of it in terms of people with learning difficulties, not just by the staff, but also by other people living with them. Some organisations are very open about any incidents of abuse, make it public and make sure it is investigated properly, but probably the small, more isolated, probably private, care homes are more high risk areas.

'The care manager, through regular visiting, isn't necessarily going to detect any sort of abuse, but what they can do is satisfy themselves that there are adequate systems and safeguards in place. The more independent people that you have got coming along, the more likely you are to discover something is going wrong.'

The importance of regular visits from social workers is illustrated perfectly by one particular case, which I looked into after it was dealt with by the Registered Homes Tribunal in December, 2000.

Alan, who has a severe learning difficulty, had been placed at a care home in Northamptonshire by Essex social services and forgotten about for over a decade.

He was eventually discovered in a locked room, unwashed and half-naked. An inspector from Northants County Council, who visited the home, described to the tribunal what he found: 'When I entered his room, [Alan] was lying curled up on a plastic-covered chair. He was wearing only a ripped tee-shirt. There was a pool of urine on the floor. The furniture in the room consisted of a wooden bed with a blue plastic mattress, a rickety table with two plastic chairs, a further plastic armchair and two wooden trunks. There was a small mat on the floor in the middle of the room, which was otherwise all lino. There was no bed linen on the bed and the room felt cold.'

A registered mental health nurse visited the same resident three months later and found him sitting unclothed in a pool of urine. She was 'very shocked' at his condition. 'When I went back one hour later there was food in Mr T's hair as well,' she told the tribunal. 'No-one had made any attempt to improve his conditions. He was sitting in the same chair, unwashed and naked. There was food in his hair and urine on the floor.'

The tribunal, which was hearing the home's appeal against the cancellation of its registration, concluded: 'The conditions in which this resident was kept were an affront to human dignity. For years, local authorities who should have been in a position to protect his human rights had ignored him and appear to have failed in their duty of care.'

The tribunal found that Alan had been kept locked in his room in 'conditions of squalor and degradation' and had been denied proper dental treatment for a painful abscess for several years. The co-owner of the home tried to explain the state of neglect by saying that 'nothing more could be done' for Alan and that he wanted to keep him 'in the same conditions in which he had been kept for the last 40 years'.

The tribunal concluded that Essex social services had 'dumped' Alan in Northants and failed to review his case properly for 12 years.

My research on this issue has not been by any means exhaustive, but, from what I have been told, I have no doubt that there are thousands of learning disabled adults in out of area placements who do not receive any visits at all from their care managers.

Because there are no statistics available, I believe there should be an independent and thorough investigation of every out-of-area placement in the country, to discover just how many vulnerable adults have been left to fend for themselves.

After all, they are at the daily mercy of the people who own and run their homes, and their staff. With no-one to complain to, they will provide perfect victims for any care workers, care managers or even fellow residents, willing to take advantage of their vulnerability. Many, hopefully, will be living in decent, pleasant homes. Many others won't.

It is a disturbing fact that many of these people—many of whom have already been damaged by decades of institutional neglect in long-stay hospitals—have been so callously cast adrift by the authorities that are supposed to be looking after them.

---

[1] David Abbott, Jenny Morris and Linda Ward: *Disabled Children and Residential Schools: A Study of Local Authority Policy and Practice*, Norah Fry Research Centre, supported by Joseph Rowntree Foundation, 2000.

AFTER LONGCARE

32. Underwhelmed

> '"Perhaps ante-natal testing should be insisted on so that Down's babies weren't born."—Comment made by a consultant obstetrician to junior doctors in the presence of a new mother.'
>
> Extract from a report on discrimination in the NHS against people with Down's Syndrome; Down's Syndrome Association; March, 1999

It was not until five or six years after that inspection unit report landed on my desk that the importance of the underwhelming reaction from the readers of the *Slough Observer* finally began to sink in.

No other conclusion could be drawn from the information I had gathered: the residents' ordeal at Longcare wasn't the fault of Gordon Rowe, or the county council staff responsible for allowing him to open Stoke Place Mansion House. It wasn't the fault of the local authorities that placed clients at the Longcare homes, either, or Slough police, the Longcare workforce, the criminal justice system, or the NHS. The more the evidence was analysed, the clearer it became who was to blame.

The residents of Longcare had been let down not by a single agency, but by every organisation which had ever come into contact with them. The abuse at Longcare was not the result of a chain of coincidences or a run of bad luck. It was born out of a systematic and deeply ingrained indifference in our society to the fate of people with learning difficulties.

And something even more disturbing slipped into place: the certainty that it would happen again.

Stoke Place and Stoke Green were scaled-down models of the Victorian and Edwardian asylums and villas for the 'mentally defective'. Their ethos was almost identical: personal possessions were discouraged, food was sparse and of poor quality, vicious punishments were administered by staff, and residents were used as indentured labour.

Rowe's regime would have concerned even the eugenicists of the early 1900s, but its principles were based on the same belief: that such people were not fit to be a part of 'normal' society.

This belief was evident in the horrified reaction of the Somerset villagers when they learned that a home for 'mentally handicapped' people was opening on their doorstep, and in the low priority accorded to learning disabled people by Buckinghamshire's social services. It was present in the police's failure to launch a proper investigation into the allegations at Longcare in 1992 and 1993, and in the care staff who failed to report Rowe's crimes. The indifference shown to the fate of learning disabled people, and the invidious belief that they should be segregated from the rest of society, were two sides of the same coin.

So have attitudes changed? Could there be another Longcare? It is easy to be reassured by listening to social services bosses who claim procedures are so much tighter now. To read the new protocol developed by Thames Valley Police for investigating abuse of vulnerable adults, and think: well, that's all sorted then. To read *Valuing People*, the government's White Paper on learning disability, and breathe a sigh of relief.

Complacency is easy. But protocols, White Papers, frameworks and taskforces achieve little on their own. The problem has always been that most people just don't care about those with learning difficulties.

They still have stones thrown through their windows, are paid derisory wages, and are denied life-saving operations by the NHS. Young men and women are still targeted by paedophiles, or forced to work for criminal gangs. Residents in care homes are still bullied, beaten, left locked up in freezing cold rooms in their own urine and faeces, and have their benefits stolen by those paid to look after them. The number of successful criminal prosecutions where the victim has a learning difficulty is still pitifully small.

Until something is done to tackle the inherent ignorance and indifference shared by the overwhelming majority of this country, people with learning difficulties will continue to live lives characterized by unhappiness and fear, just as they did at Longcare.

33. 'You Couldn't Hear Anyone Coming'

> 'If you are told what to do all the time you forget how to make your own decisions,' said Kay. 'You lose your self respect. But once you start making your own decisions life just gets better and better.'
>
> Kay Warren, a woman with a learning difficulty and a volunteer with Skills for People, interviewed in the *Evening Chronicle*, Newcastle, January 29, 2001

Many people believe that it doesn't much matter if you hurt someone with a learning difficulty, because 'they don't have feelings like normal people'. The psychotherapists who work for Respond know differently. In the months and years after the abuse at Longcare was first revealed, it was Respond which provided counselling for many of Gordon Rowe's victims.

In the wake of the first newspaper reports, Respond started to receive requests for help from local authorities who wanted to know if their clients had been abused, and whether they should be moved to new homes. The charity's work was vital in convincing many councils to move their clients away from Longcare as quickly as possible.

As residents began to leave, the care workers in their new homes started to notice worrying signs of trauma. By November, 1994, Respond was receiving the first in a new wave of inquiries. This time, they were being asked to provide treatment. By Christmas of that year, they were holding their first counselling sessions.

Not all of the victims Respond treated had been beaten or raped by Gordon Rowe. Many were suffering from the effects of living for many years in an atmosphere of cruelty and inhumanity, and witnessing assaults taking place around them.

'Sexual abuse is always what catches people's imagination,' Philippa Russell told me, 'but sexual abuse is part of a wider pattern of abuse. Adults who have been sexually abused have almost invariably been emotionally abused and physically abused in a whole variety of ways. In many ways the most shocking thing about Longcare was the persistence, the day to day cruelty.

'One of the women... was regularly slammed outside in her chair to sit outside in the rain, the sleet and the snow, if she didn't eat properly or talked at mealtimes. If she hears a voice raised now, she'll grab a chair and bolt for the door.'

Russell, who is herself the mother of son with a learning difficulty, remembers being shown around Stoke Place by a resident, during one of the visits by the inquiry team. Once Longcare had gone, the house was 'actually quite nice', she told me. 'But it was creepy to walk through the private part of the house, where the bedrooms were. There was a beautiful, large sitting-room on the first floor, looking down the park, and the residents wouldn't go into this beautiful room, which was furnished, and carpeted, with pictures, because that is where so much of the abuse took place. Even more horribly, when you walked into this part of the building, you couldn't hear anything. It was all muffled and dull, because of this really thick shag-pile carpet, which in some cases extended up like a sort of dado. A resident said to me, absolutely clearly, with a straight face, 'well, of course, you couldn't hear anyone coming. You didn't want to go to sleep at night.' It shows you how awful it really was.'

Many former Longcare residents counselled by Respond were desperately frightened and anxious. In one of them, this showed itself through a phobia of birds. Even the sight of a bird drawn on a piece of paper was enough to spark screaming panic. Many shared an 'abnormal' fear of authority and were almost pathologically incapable of disobedience. If another person entered the room, they would cower in the corner. They were jumpy, constantly looking around for signs of danger. Many also had eating disorders, or found it impossible to enjoy a full night's sleep without the interruption of nightmares. Others couldn't sleep at all without the light left on, and some were too frightened to go into a bathroom to take a bath.

As these men and women began courses of long-term psychotherapy, a number of similar symptoms began to emerge: depression, low self-esteem and an inability to express emotions such as joy, sadness, or anger. They were showing classic symptoms of post-traumatic stress disorder.

'There is no reason at all why someone with a learning disability should display signs of post-traumatic stress disorder,' Alan Corbett told me. 'Nor did we find people were suffering from psychosis or other forms of mental illness. These were people who clearly showed signs of being traumatised over a long period of time.'

The central problem in treating people with severe learning difficulties is how to communicate with them. Many of the Longcare victims could only speak a few words. Corbett told me: 'Although the inability to speak may make therapy and counselling a longer and more difficult process, it does not mean that therapy or counselling cannot be used at all. Respond has learned that people who lack verbal skills learn to communicate in many other ways. You can tell someone is clinically depressed by their posture, by how they move, by observing them. If someone is banging her head against the wall, or rocking violently, or cutting her arm, or throwing herself on the floor, those are powerful connections with something that has been done that cannot be put into words.'

Corbett believes society has made people with learning difficulties 'a very vulnerable group'. 'They are perfect victims, ready for the picking. We have been denying that people with learning difficulties are different, but they do have difficulties that make them vulnerable and we should not delude ourselves that they do not. The extent and practice of sexual abuse should be recognised rather than denied.'

In the spring of 2001, I spoke to Corbett again. He told me the charity had eventually counselled about 10 former Longcare clients. Respond was still in contact with these victims and those who were now looking after them. But there were no miracle cures for Rowe's victims. None of them 'got better'.

'What therapy was able to provide the victims of Longcare was a space in which they were believed and a space in which their experiences could be processed,' says Corbett. 'What it didn't remove was the terrible reality of those experiences. We were able to provide people with relief from much of the pain of what they had gone through, but when you think of the enormity of the damage, you have to think about a long-term therapeutic plan. For these victims, probably for years and years, people will have to think about their care in a different way.'

They will have to cope with feelings of fear, guilt and shame they will never lose, he said. 'Therapy can help enormously with much of that, but given the severity of the damage, it is not going to stop all of the pain.'

In the autumn of 2002, Corbett told me about a new client, another former Longcare resident who had only recently been put in touch with Respond. Although his social services department had lost all his personal records, the man's new case worker had managed to piece together a picture of his history. He has talked about being shouted at and kicked at Longcare and having his hair pulled. He is also believed to have been sexually abused by Gordon Rowe. He has various eating disorders, paranoia and a fear of men. He spends all day locked in his room, watching television with the sound turned down. If he hears a sudden noise, he will immediately 'retreat into himself'. There are serious concerns about his weight, says Corbett. He seems to be just wasting away.

In May 2003, I was handed further confirmation of the devastating long-term consequences of the Longcare abuse. Ali O'Callaghan and Professor Glynis Murphy of The Tizard Centre at the University of Kent and Dr Isabel Clare of Cambridge University's Department of Psychiatry had been researching the effects of long-term abuse on severely learning disabled people, with funding from the Department of Health. They had talked to the families of eighteen, mostly young, men and women who had been abused. Many had been Longcare residents.

I was handed a summary of the new and as yet unpublished research. It showed the victims had suffered 'significant psychological distress' immediately after the abuse, with behavioural problems, self-harm and sleep problems. Although, with time, there had been 'some alleviation in the frequency and severity of this distress... not one person had recovered completely'. The research also talked about the guilt, depression and inability to trust care workers felt by the families.

'At present,' they concluded, 'there seems to be little recognition of the serious and long-term impact of abuse on both people with learning disabilities and those who care about them.'

Philippa Russell came across one more piece of disturbing evidence during her visit to Longcare. She was told by a number of people that Gordon Rowe had been running a prostitution ring out of Stoke Place.

'I'm not saying I have evidence that there was an organised prostitution racket. But Gordon Rowe knew a lot of people. Presumably, one doesn't know how, this whole thing was connected up. You couldn't prove any of these things, but the allegations are such that clearly something happened. We had this from ex-members of staff, but we were also told it by a number of people from local voluntary organisations.'

'Of course, these rumours can roll like snowballs,' says Russell. 'All one can say is that there were worrying allegations and it seems extremely unlikely that there was not a strong element of truth, about people coming into the house in the evening. A lot of the residents were clear that there were strangers, and some of the younger women say they were taken out of the house.

'I heard quite a lot about the 'people in the night', because of talking to [residents] in their rooms. I was told how pleased everybody was to have locks put on their doors. They were really worried at night. There was a dog living there and one man said to me that he used to encourage the dog to sleep in his room at night, because then if anybody came in, the dog would immediately jump up.'

Russell believes the prostitution ring links up with Rowe's filmmaking hobby, and the suspicion that he was making and selling pornographic videos. 'It is unthinkable actually that these things weren't going on, knowing what one knows about... Rowe's interests.

'I should think Gordon Rowe was engaged with a lot of other people, and that there are a fair number of people down in Buckinghamshire who are still a bit shaky about what might come out.'

34. 'I Want Something Better'

> 'If every person with a learning difficulty across the country was part of a self-advocacy group, then that would send a message to social service professionals who think they know it all.'
>
> Andrew Lee, director of London People First, quoted in *The Guardian*, April 14, 2001

I had heard a lot about People First, an umbrella organisation of loosely affiliated groups whose members offer help and advice to people with learning difficulties. But there the similarities with most other such groups end, because People First is also run by people with learning difficulties. They are helped by non-disabled supporters, who are there to offer assistance, if needed. But these supporters take a passive role, giving advice only when asked.

Members of People First believe in self-advocacy, the idea that people with learning difficulties are the ones best qualified to improve the quality of their own lives, rather than leaving it to the 'professionals'—the social workers and the care assistants. But they also act as advocates themselves to other people with learning difficulties who need support.

I arranged to meet four members of the Central England branch of People First: Ian Davies, Janet Pheasant, Nigel Lott and Craig Hart.

When I arrived in the road in which their headquarters are based, I could not find their offices, so I asked a passing resident. She had never heard of People First. I finally found their front door, marked clearly with a 'People First' sign, directly across the road from where I had approached the woman. I looked back across the road and she smiled and shrugged her shoulders. 'I never noticed it before,' she said.

The bell wasn't working, so I knocked on the door. It was answered by Ian Davies, one of the founders of the Central England branch of People First. He introduced himself and invited me in. Inside, I met the other members of the team, working at their computers in the main office. The surroundings had an air of casual neglect, a contrast to the industry practised by the volunteers.

After the introductions, we moved down the corridor to another dusty room and sat in a rough circle: myself, Janet on my left, then Neil Morris, a softly-spoken Kiwi, the supporter, who was there to offer assistance if needed. Next to him was Nigel, the only married member of the quartet, who has been involved in the group from its early days, Craig, and Ian.

At several points during the two-hour discussion that followed, members of the group left the room without warning or explanation. Particularly Janet. One of her colleagues explained that she had a short attention span. I later discovered that she had made herself a cup of tea and had then been distracted by a phone call and decided to do some work on her computer. After some initial shyness, I found all four of them bright and insightful. Some of their comments surprised and even shocked me. Although they sometimes took a while to understand a question, at no point did I feel that they were confused or unable to grasp the issues.

Ian told me the group started ten years ago. 'Everyone in this room, everyone here was in day services, in residential care homes. At that time it was always dominated by professionals. Staff, researchers, health authority, care managers. The problem we were having is our ideas were being dictated by these people. We didn't have a voice of our own. It had always been dominated by the professionals. There was a bit of resistance from a lot of people regarding People First. A lot of people. All the regular authorities from social services down to day service managers. They were thinking we couldn't run our own organisation, we couldn't be our own bosses. They didn't think we could do things for ourselves. They wanted to hold all the purse strings. We have proved them wrong.'

'We are our own boss,' Janet added. 'We can make our own choices. There is one thing we do not like. That's being given as a label.'

'People First has a saying,' said Nigel. 'Label Jars, Not People.'

I asked whether any of them had experienced discrimination or abuse. Yes, said Ian. 'They see something, they just want to make a meal of it. Spastic, four eyes, all those sort of labels, and a lot of that is from the general public. If they were to educate their children in a better sense and direction then the children of today would not be thinking the same way as their parents would.'

'People walk past, looking at you,' said Craig. A few minutes later, he adds: 'I had one last month. I reported it, but since then… I reported it to the police. They have not found any clues. They do not know if it's him or not. I feel angry since after that. He punched me in the face. Just feel like a bit bored or might be a bit drunk. I just said to a friend he might come back and do it again. I feel angry and I just feel being on my own.'

Janet told me how the group aims to help other people with learning difficulties. 'If that person has a learning difficulty and they are finding it hard to speak up for themselves, that's where we come in, we can talk to them and speak up for them. Sometimes they can turn to us if they want to talk to us for help. I am in the process of working with a young lady. Without going into too many details, I feel very strongly about it…'

I asked them why advocacy was so important. 'I think it is important so we know how they feel,' said Nigel. 'It's their choice. It's their home. They should be saying what they want and what they want to do in it.'

I met Neil Morris later again by accident. He said the group could have told me far more than they had. It was a question of trust. They had only just met me and I was a journalist. Some of their personal experiences of discrimination and harassment were horrific, he said.

The conversation reminded me of what I had been told by former members of Longcare staff. How residents had taken months to trust care workers enough to confide in them. This question of trust was forced home to me when I received an email from Ian Davies the day after my visit:

Hi John
We found the meeting useful. We look forward to reading the book. We just want to remind you that it is important to use our

words and to give us credit for the things we said. While respecting the confidentiality we requested.

Hope your book helps to change things.

Cheers,
Ian Davies

People First believe that self-advocacy and the use of advocates who themselves have learning difficulties are crucial defences against abuse.

People with learning difficulties seem to find it much easier to trust someone else with a similar disability, rather than a 'professional'. They instinctively distrust professionals—whether social workers, lawyers, health managers or police officers. They hate being talked down to. They want to take the initiative. They do not like to be ignored and patronised.

The self-advocacy movement is about enabling those people without a voice to speak up for themselves. It is about helping people to find a voice, and to use it. The self-advocacy movement is never going to eradicate abuse. But it is a powerful tool for tackling the problem, because it is about encouraging victims to speak out. And once that silence is broken, the other difficulties they face become less daunting.

I was honoured to be the only journalist invited to cover Central England People First's conference on the *Valuing People* White Paper in the autumn of 2001. Apart from me, the only people allowed to attend were those with learning difficulties and their supporters. It didn't run like clockwork, but it worked. And scores of people with learning difficulties stood up on stage to have their say about the issues that affected their lives. It was, even for a journalist, an inspiring experience, and it showed that the self-advocacy movement has huge potential for improving the lives of people with learning difficulties.

There are signs that People First and similar organisations around the world are making progress. The growing use of the internet by members of self-advocacy organisations to share ideas and news is one encouraging development.

If every residential home and day service in the country was forced to set up self-advocacy groups, with staff banned from meetings, how much greater would be the chance of alerting those who need to know about bullying, brutality and abuse?

But the self-advocacy movement will not have an easy ride. There is a wall of cynicism to breach, but also the suspicion that self-advocacy benefits those with milder learning difficulties much more than it does those with more profound disabilities. Its supporters have had to fight for the ground they have won.

A good friend, Lisa Sherper, who lives in the United States, described the reaction of many of the people she tried to talk to about the subject of this book. She said they were often disturbed by the subject matter and unwilling to discuss it.

Many people still feel deeply uneasy about people with learning difficulties. They often turn away, whether from day-to-day contact or discussion of issues such as abuse. This is deeply worrying, because without increased public awareness, potential abusers will find it much easier to escape detection and justice.

The abuse of people with learning difficulties has always gone on. The institutionalisation of care in the nineteenth and early twentieth centuries provided bullies and abusers with easy access to potential victims. The possibility that such abuse is a late twentieth century phenomenon is not very credible. The truth is that idiots/the mentally defective/the mentally subnormal/the mentally handicapped/people with learning disabilities/people with learning difficulties have always provided easy targets for those willing to take advantage of their vulnerability.

Training, awareness campaigns, *Valuing People*, anti-harassment policies, advocacy projects, new legislation on care standards, new sexual offences legislation and legislation on evidence. All these measures seem to have one factor in common: the need for better communication. And the best way that can be achieved is by trying to change some very deep-rooted discrimination and prejudice. Without a shift in attitudes, people with learning difficulties will remain on the outskirts of society, stared at but not talked to, and denied the opportunity for interaction that might allow them to reveal a concern, a fear, or a crime. There is no chance that such measures will eradicate the sexual, physical, emotional, verbal and financial abuse of people with learning difficulties. There are too many reasons why such crimes may stay hidden. But nothing would make the detection and prevention of abuse more likely than the development of friendships between people with, and people without, learning difficulties.

A simple starting point would be at least to give proper support to organisations such as People First, and recognise the strength of their initiative.

35. Ninety Per Cent

> 'In fifty years' time, self advocates imagine a world in which people with learning difficulties live independently, earn money, get married, have children. A world in which they are free from harassment and abuse. They can see a future in which People First will be Britain's 'principal pressure group for people with a learning disability'. When the government's minister for disabled people will have learning difficulties.'
>
> Excerpt from article by Tara Mack, *The Guardian*, April 14, 2001

A survey by Mencap (*Living in Fear*, June 1999) found that two-thirds of people with a learning difficulty were bullied at least once a month, whether through name-calling, harassment, threats, or physical assaults. Nearly ninety per cent had been bullied in the previous year.

The survey quoted one Glasgow woman, aged forty, who said: 'I get called stupid, teased all the time. Children follow me every day and call me names, threaten to kill me, in the street and at the centre.'

Name-calling often escalates to something more serious, as the perpetrators realise they can get away with offences against a learning disabled person. Most incidents are totally unprovoked. They can occur anywhere: at a bus stop, in the street, in public leisure facilities, shops, pubs, even in people's own homes.

Mencap's survey was backed up in the autumn of 2002, when the crime reduction charity NACRO reported that nine out of ten people with learning difficulties questioned for its research[1] had been verbally harassed in the previous year. The report found that disabled people as a whole were four times more likely to be violently assaulted than non-disabled people and four times more likely to be sexually assaulted, but were less likely to report offences and were not taken seriously enough when they did. Procedures for reporting crime and providing witness statements did not take the needs of people with learning difficulties into account, said the report, published more than eight years after the failures of Thames Valley Police were exposed by the Longcare abuse.

Ill-treatment in health settings has not disappeared, either. In 1997, an external review panel was set up to examine Community Health Care: North Durham NHS Trust, in the wake of the death of one patient with a learning difficulty and the serious injury of another in road traffic accidents.

The following year, the panel reported how an internal investigation at the trust had led to a series of serious allegations. Patients had been frog-marched by staff, others were 'secluded' in toilets, one was put in a cold bath, and there was a 'failure to abide by drug administration procedures' and to 'adhere to professional nursing codes of conduct'.

These were the kind of concerns raised during the long-stay hospital scandals of the 60s and 70s.

In the summer of 2001, Mencap reported that a survey had uncovered worrying evidence of the abuse of disabled people's human rights within the NHS.

In one case, medical staff placed a 'do not resuscitate' notice on the records of a 24-year-old woman with learning and physical disabilities, who had developed a serious respiratory infection, without telling her parents. She was refused intensive care and her parents were told that she could not be placed on a life support machine because of her 'age, disability, quality of life and the cost'. She died. Her father believes doctors allowed her to die because of her disabilities.

Mencap collected many other examples of such discrimination. Often they involved medical staff placing 'do not resuscitate' notices on patient records, or judges deciding that lives were 'not worth living'.

Of course, medical staff need better training. But the survey showed that many GPs, dentists, nurses, opticians and paediatricians hold the same views about people with learning difficulties as most of the rest of the population: they see them as second-, third- or even fourth-class citizens.

One piece of research illustrated how urgently change is needed. Dr Dinah K C Murray described how tens of thousands of learning disabled people were on repeat prescriptions of anti-psychotic drugs, which can have devastating effects on their bodies.[2] The list of potential side-effects includes: difficulty talking, urinating and swallowing, fatigue, jerky movements of head, face, mouth or neck, drooling saliva, skin rashes, sore throat, swelling of feet, trembling of hands, uncontrollable lip movements and weight gain. The drugs—which include some of those prescribed for the Longcare residents, such as Largactil—can also cause sudden death.

These drugs are often used as tranquillisers, as Rowe used them, or to calm behaviours that might annoy or alarm other people, such as anger, frustration or shouting, in the mistaken belief that they are actually showing symptoms of psychosis.

Murray's research shows a frightening tendency among professionals—particularly GPs and care workers—to simply reach for the drugs when confronted with behaviour they don't understand or don't want to understand. The overuse of neuroleptic drugs is a form of abuse. It is rooted, just as other abuse and discrimination is, in the failure to recognise the person behind the disability.

But what about the kind of institutional abuse witnessed at Longcare? Has that been eradicated?

Not according to Nick Johnson, assistant chief executive of the Social Care Association, which represents care workers. He believes there are more such cases to come. 'I think there will be more than that one,' he told me. 'I do not think that was the end of it. There are individuals who are in trouble as I speak.'

In April, 2002, I gave a talk about the Longcare case to a network of adult protection managers. They were responsible for co-ordinating investigations into alleged abuse of adults with learning difficulties, and other vulnerable groups. I had expected them to tell me that cases of institutional abuse had been almost eliminated by the new legislation and adult protection systems now in place. But, instead, they told me of new cases, new investigations, and widespread suspected abuse and bad practice. Eight years on from Longcare, there was no sign that the institutional abuse of learning disabled people was any less common than it had ever been.

As for sexual abuse, few cases ever reach the courts. Often, a successful prosecution is only possible because the offender has been careless. The cunning ones, like Rowe, are still able to escape justice. One who *was* successfully convicted was agency care worker Phillip Kambeta, who raped a 24-year-old woman with severe learning difficulties at a Nottingham care home, after using another man's national insurance number to secure his job. Kambeta, who was eventually sentenced to 12 years in prison, was only found out because he made the woman pregnant.

In November, 1999, the charity Respond set up a help-line for people who wanted to report or discuss abuse of people with learning difficulties. By the autumn of 2002, calls to the help-line had risen from 500 a year to 1,100 a year. Most were allegations of abuse.

Alan Corbett is head of clinical services at the charity, which offers psychotherapy and counselling to learning disabled people who have been abused. He says the helpline receives many calls from mothers who 'find themselves faced with a system that doesn't seem to hear them'.

'They are ringing in about their children, who have been abused, often over periods of years, but certainly no legal justice has been undertaken and no therapeutic justice either. This is happening across the board—residential, special schools, day centres. Anywhere where people with learning disabilities congregate. We seem to be hearing a worrying number of cases of abuse, deprivation and neglect.'

Corbett said Respond was 'working with more people than we ever have before', with an increasing number of calls about learning disabled children. 'We deal with all aspects of abuse—sexual, physical, emotional—but the majority of people who come through the doors have been sexually abused. What we are finding is that we are being asked to work more with people who are clearly traumatised in all kinds of ways. Something terrible has happened to them, but nobody knows quite what. Often that something terrible may be rooted in very early childhood experience. If you are working with someone who lacks words to describe that, you may never know what that is.'

Experts are convinced that paedophiles are now targeting young people with learning difficulties as they find themselves frustrated by the tightening of legislation and increased public awareness in their attempts to gain access to non-disabled children.

An NSPCC spokeswoman told me in 2001: 'It is horrible to think that these young people, who have enough to face in their lives as it is, could become targets for paedophiles. It does happen, and the trouble is that sometimes they cannot communicate when it does happen. I think if the genuine figures were known it would be shocking.'

What is most shocking, of course, is that the vast majority of cases of abuse never even result in a complaint to the police, let alone a criminal conviction.

Research by Michelle McCarthy and David Thompson[3] suggested that as many as 61 per cent of women and 25 per cent of men with learning difficulties had been sexually abused. Earlier, unpublished, research quoted in their study had found as many as 83 per cent of users of a day service had been abused.

When the problem is so vast, so overpowering, it is unlikely that any measures to tackle discrimination in the legal system and poor standards in the care system can do anything but make a small dent in what is nothing short of an appalling epidemic of sexual, and physical, victimisation.

[1] Samantha Cunningham and Susannah Drury, *Access all Areas*, NACRO; 2002.
[2] Dr Dinah K C Murray; *Potions, Pills and Community Care for People with Learning Difficulties: Hidden Costs*; May 1999
[3] Michelle McCarthy and David Thompson, *A Prevalence Study of Sexual Abuse of Adults with Intellectual Disabilities Referred for Sex Education; Journal of Applied Research in Intellectual Disabilities*, Vol 10, No 2, 1997

36. Dorothy

'Southwark Council in south London has apologised unreservedly for the physical abuse and neglect of a woman in its care who has a severe learning disability, is blind, has partial hearing and almost no speech. The move follows a damning report by the local government ombudsman, who found the authority guilty of maladministration causing injustice over the care of the thirty-nine-year-old woman, who is not identified. "Among other things," reports the ombudsman, Edward Osmotherly, "she was assaulted twice by staff, she sustained many injuries (including a fractured skull) and I am not satisfied that her medication was properly administered. It took too long for the council to move her to another place, which would be suitable for her".'

The Guardian, 'Society' section; July 18, 2001

Most of the Longcare residents are not able to talk about their experiences at Stoke Place and Stoke Green, although some have been able to give their relatives a vague idea of what it was like: a half-remembered phrase here, a fragment of an episode there.

But Dorothy Thomson, one of the most able of his victims is one former Longcare resident who has been able to give a detailed and damning description of life under Gordon Rowe and how she coped afterwards.

I first spoke to Dorothy a few days before New Year's Eve, 1999, at her home in Hampshire. Dorothy survived Botley's Park and Stoke Place by clinging onto a 'dream' that one day she would have a flat of her own and would be able to 'settle down'. She now shares a flat in a sheltered development with her husband Jamie. Jamie is in his early forties. He had brain damage as a five-year-old, after contracting meningitis, and takes medication for epilepsy.

Dorothy always vowed that if she married, it would be to a disabled man who needed help and 'guidance for living out in the community'. She sees that as part of her role, now. 'Nothing else matters to me, only Jamie. He's the only one that's really respected me and I have given him my love, too. The fear is there that if anything happened to Jamie, what am I going to do?'

The shelves of Dorothy and Jamie's living room are covered with porcelain dolls. Dorothy has more than fifty in her collection. There are dolls dressed as nuns, others in Edwardian costumes. 'To me, everything in here is sort of alive,' she says. 'It's not sort of cold and dead.' The dolls and the soft toys in her bedroom are reminders of a childhood she was never allowed to enjoy.

One of the things she values most of all now is her independence. At Longcare, Gordon Rowe decided at what time the residents should eat and how they would spend every minute of their days. If they didn't conform to the regime, they were punished. 'If you wasn't down on time for breakfast, you was hungry for the rest of the day, so time is a big asset.'

But even though Dorothy has married and settled down, she still has to confront every day the reality of what it is like to have a learning difficulty in the 21st century.

'Even now I worry about Jamie. If he goes out for long periods, what'll happen to him? Because I know best of all what the world is like towards disabled people. Even [if] we both go out now we both get insulted, but I taught Jamie not to say anything, so he doesn't. But that doesn't leave the fear inside of you when he goes out. It's always going to be there, that fear. Even if I married somebody body abled, that fear would still be there. That's why I tell him off sometimes, because the fear is there.'

Her experiences have also given her what she calls 'that bitter tinge of life', but also the strength and obstinacy so that 'if anybody says anything or does anything then I will not hesitate to hit back'.

Her exposure to life in the long-stay wards of Botley's Park and under the brutal regime of Gordon Rowe has also made her a more caring person. 'If I go out now and see somebody beating someone up, I wouldn't hesitate to intervene.' Only that morning, she had been helping a new neighbour settle into her flat, Dorothy's social worker told me. She also donates money to the Blue Cross animal charity and performs voluntary work for the cerebral palsy charity Scope. 'If it was up to me, I would actually work in a mental home,' she says. She has offered to have former Longcare residents to stay in her flat on holiday.

The abusive regime run by Gordon Rowe drove Dorothy deep into depression. 'I was very suicidal for about two or three years. I used to try and make suicide. When I went to bed, I used to put needles down my arms just so that I could drip blood just like a doctor. I used to hoard tablets up and take then and make myself pretty ill, because the treatment there, you couldn't visualise it being inflicted on a human. I used to say to look at my life just pick up a horror movie, the worst one, and put it in, and you could see my life in reflection.'

'I feel sorry for the rest of the residents that are living,' she says, 'because they can't talk about it and the scars are right there. What was annoying is that Gordon Rowe thought that they wouldn't hurt or anything, but they used to come to me and say how much they were hurting. A lot of them would tell me that they were fed up with life and I used to coax them to get on with it and not take any notice. It was my sense of humour that brought them through it in the end.'

Christianity was one of the factors that helped Dorothy through her ordeal. 'I've got a very big faith, so strong. I think that's what gives me the energy. I mean, even though—you might not understand this bit—they did cruel things to me, Gordon Rowe and Angela Rowe and Nigel Rowe and that, but then if they came to this front door and they said, "Oh, hello Dorothy, how are you?" I would say, "Do you want to come in for a cup of tea, Angela Rowe?" I would, yes, because isn't that what Christianity is about—forgiveness?'

Her experiences have convinced her that society must change how it treats disabled people. 'I think it's about time people started coming out of the Middle Ages and respecting the disabled people, not going round making fun of them, not laughing at them, but showing them a little bit of compassion, because who knows what that disabled person goes through? Who knows they are not going to have a child that will end up the same?'

Dorothy's years in Stoke Place have also had a lasting impact on how she reacts to seemingly normal situations.

'It takes a hell of a lot for me to trust anybody now,' she says. 'I won't even trust the wardens. I can't go to a doctors if I was ill.' It has also damaged her ability to react to stress and pain in a normal way. 'I broke my arm once. I fell on the floor in Stoke Place. I just laughed, because that's the only way that I can beat pain. If you cried [at Stoke Place] you got punished. If you didn't stop crying, you got punished.

'I cannot go into a room now that is crowded or has a party.' Residents were forced to attend parties and put smiles on their faces and 'enjoy' themselves. 'If you didn't go, you had very bad punishments inflicted on you. And if you didn't smile, you had to smile. That's why I'm always laughing now, even when I've hurt myself. To me, life is a joke, and I see it that way. That's the life I was brought up into, the life of a joke.'

I ask her what she hated most about Stoke Place. 'You couldn't have a meal in peace, you couldn't sleep in peace, you couldn't go to your room to have a quiet sit down, because Gordon Rowe had them all rigged up with intercoms and he wanted to know who was in your room and what you were saying.'

She also remembers how Gordon and another employee of Longcare would 'play around with your feelings'. This woman, she says, used to call Jimmy over at mealtimes and give him extra food, and then 'kiss and fondle him'. 'She would also do the same with David. He would lay down and she was stride over him sort of hitting him, and she would say, "well, David, would you like to be whipped?" She never knew that I knew what it all meant.'

Gordon took every possible opportunity to try to break Dorothy's spirit. 'He would just attack me by saying, "you can't have any tea because of doing this", or he would say, "go upstairs, you're not to have nothing".' He also nicknamed her 'Dysentery'. Dorothy knew exactly what it meant.

Rowe knew the important things in his residents' lives. In Dorothy's case, he knew how much she loved Jimmy, her boyfriend. So he split them up and sent Dorothy back from the gatehouse to live at Stoke Place for six months. Dorothy believes this was because she had tried to help other residents. 'Gordon Rowe took me back to Stoke Place and left Jimmy in the group home and I just banged my head on the toilet on the shower room. I just wanted to crush my own brains in. I couldn't stand the hurt anymore. Yeah, I wanted to crush my own skull in. He was a very devious, cruel man.'

She still thinks about Gordon Rowe, and about Angela, and of the 'innocent blood' that is on their hands. 'All Angela Rowe got was two and a half years. But how many years did she give the disabled, how many years of agony, corruption, cruelty, agonising torture?'

But Dorothy says she is most angry with the legal system that allowed Rowe, Desmond Tully and Lorraine Field to get away with such light sentences. 'I'm not angry with Stoke Place, I'm angry with people, I'm angry with the Government, I'm angry with the courts.'

37. Rosie

> 'Liz Peters is holding her comfort cat toy as she tells her story. She is twenty two and has Downs syndrome...Sitting with her parents, Ms Peters is comfortable with what she is saying but it took a long time to achieve that. 'He had sex on me. He touched my boobs and bottom—don't like it. I told him no, but he just kept doing it. I never told anybody what happened because he said 'Don't tell your mummy and daddy or the police'. He was just naughty. He had sex on me in the laundry room and nobody saw me.' Ms Peters was abused systematically by a care worker in the home where she had lived for a number of years.'
>
> The Guardian, September 17, 2001

Benedict Alcindor: 'When I telephoned Rosie, she would often say she wanted to come home. I told her we would visit her more often. When she did come home for a visit, she never wanted to go back. When it was time to return to Longcare, her face changed and she would make herself sick.'

It is a late summer day in Benedict's flat in Tower Hamlets, east London. We are talking in the living-room, surrounded by pictures of her large family. 'I figured maybe she was just missing the family, that she wasn't seeing enough of us,' she tells me. 'Then, one Christmas, she gathered all her dolls together and asked me to take them home for her.'

On visits home, Rosie would often touch her belly and tell her aunt that it hurt. Benedict would give her a kiss and a few comforting words. And there were the stitches in an ankle wound Rosie blamed on a fall against a radiator. And the birth control pills Rowe said were to control her periods and 'stop the blood clotting'.

Like most of the Longcare relatives, the first Benedict knew of the lengthy investigation Bucks County Council had conducted was through television news coverage of the stories the *Slough Observer* and *The Independent* had run about the leaked report. She was shocked, but never for a moment believed Rosie was one of those affected. She rang Tower Hamlets, her local authority, and nothing she was told made her believe anything different.

A few weeks later, Rosie was rushed into Slough's Wexham Park Hospital. She had had a severe epileptic seizure and the hospital was not sure she would pull through. After one visit, Rosie's social worker told Benedict she believed Rosie had been abused. 'I couldn't believe her. I couldn't believe she was one of them,' Benedict tells me.

The family were already looking for a new place for Rosie to live, and in February, 1995, she moved to a small home in east London, nearer Benedict's home. A few weeks later, Rosie came home to celebrate Mother's Day. It was a weekend Benedict would never forget.

She was cooking in the kitchen on the Saturday afternoon, cleaning some chicken, ready for a big family meal the next day, when Rosie walked into the room, asked what she was doing and pointed to her belly, as she had done several times before. She told her aunt it was hurting. Then she said: 'He nearly kill me.'

'Who?' asked Benedict.

'Big Dada,' said Rosie.

'What happened?' asked her aunt. Appalled, she watched as her niece bunched her fingers, performed an unmistakable action with her fist, and pointed to her genitals.

'He nearly kill me,' she repeated.

'Where did it happen?'

'In my room.'

'Who was with you?'

'Only two of us. He put me down on floor. He nearly kill me. He drink milk,' she said, and pointed to her breasts. Then she described how the same thing had happened at the cottage.

'Where was Big Mama?' asked Benedict.

'She wasn't there,' replied Rosie. 'She went shopping.'

'Where was Baby Ben?'

'He wasn't there. He went shopping with Big Mama. He put me on the floor. He nearly kill me.'

The next day, Mother's Day, Rosie joined the rest of the family in church. 'She was standing next to me as we were singing a hymn and the words were so right that the tears were coming down,' says Benedict. 'Rosie looked at me and said, "Mama, you're crying." I was just a wreck.'

Later, Rosie said she was also going to tell her brothers and sisters. 'We were all sitting round the table having dinner and she explained to all of us what happened,' says Benedict. 'It was so sad.'

'I was just like a crazy person. I didn't want to believe what she had told me, that she was one of them,' says Benedict. 'I trusted that man so much because he was like a father to her.'

The shock hurt her so badly that her family had to send her away for a holiday. But it didn't work. 'I was crying. My heart was bleeding. I lost weight. I couldn't eat. I couldn't sleep. It was like there was a big brick in my heart that I couldn't get out.'

Her first husband died on the operating table. The pain was terrible, but she pulled through and eventually remarried. This was different, she says. It is a pain that has yet to fade, and shows no sign that it ever will.

'It has just finished me. For the kid to be there for ten years. Damaging her, damaging me. I blame myself. If I had taken any notice of her…she was already damaged, but maybe… Now the more it carries on, the more it hurts me. The feeling is eating me. The way she said it all innocently: "He nearly kill me. He nearly kill me."'

When I next speak to Benedict, three years later, in the early summer of 2001, I hope this pain has faded. But, if anything, it has grown more intense.

As if the family had not had enough to cope with, another of Benedict's nieces has recently been beaten to death in London. Benedict's brother returned from St Lucia to bury his daughter and died suddenly the next day. The family held a double funeral. Benedict has had her own health problems, undergoing an operation on her spine.

Guilt is still gnawing at her. 'Each time I look at her picture, it is a pain in my heart that is damaging me, eating me up,' she says.

As she talks to me on the telephone, Benedict cries quietly. 'It has damaged my life. I can't smile, because I blame my own self. Each time she said she was not going back and she was bringing her dolls and showing her feeling and saying it was hurting, and I didn't take any notice. I thought that she saw my children and wanted to stay home. I didn't want to listen to her, thinking she was playing up… It is doing my head, it is doing my brain, my heart, the burning, the pain, it doesn't go away. I need to move on, but it doesn't feel like I am moving on. All the pain is there, the pressure, the hurt, it is like a lump, something that needs to come out.'

Rosie likes to sing and dance and hates to cause problems for others. She can make a cup of tea and put her own clothes on and is clean and tidy.

'She is a nice kid,' says her aunt, 'a happy-going girl. She's not stupid either. She's a clever girl.' Rosie knows Rowe is dead, but the merest reminder of him or Stoke Place is enough to cause an epileptic seizure.

'She spent ten years of her life there. At the end, she said nobody loved her no more. Big Dada and Big Mama didn't love her no more. I knew Angela was a bit rough, but I always thought Rowe was nice. I couldn't see that he would do anything wrong, that he would take advantage of them.'

Rosie was visited three or four times at Longcare by her social worker in her first year there, but after that he left Tower Hamlets and wasn't replaced. 'I was doing all the running, all the chasing, all the visiting,' says Benedict, 'but I didn't have the knowledge to ask the questions.'

38. Greg

'A TV gardener who indecently assaulted a young man with a learning disability has been jailed for two and a half years. Dennis Cornish, sixty one, Carlton West Country's TV gardener, was found guilty of two assaults. His victim had been taking part in a horticultural training project next to Cornish's garden centre in Stoke Gabriel, Devon.'

Disability Now, July, 2000

When Gordon Rowe left The Old Rectory in Somerset, Norma Adams assumed her complaints had been investigated by the authorities and proven unfounded.

Within a few weeks of his departure, the new management at The Old Rectory asked Norma to find Greg a new home. He had become unmanageable and aggressive and the staff decided they could no longer cope.

Norma agreed to have Greg temporarily admitted to Leavesden Hospital near Watford. She was ill with suspected colonic cancer and it was three weeks before she was fit enough to visit. When she arrived, one of the nurses told her: 'I don't understand what this is all about. Greg is here with a record of aggression, but he is such a sweetie.' Norma believes the heavy use of tranquillisers at The Old Rectory caused the aggression. Once Greg was taken off the drugs, the belligerence vanished.

Ten years later, Greg had settled into a new home. His mother believed he was finally content and stable, and The Old Rectory was a fading memory. That was until she turned on the news one evening and saw a story about Gordon Rowe and Stoke Place. She was appalled, and contacted Slough police. She was assured they already knew about The Old Rectory. Of course they did. Everybody knew.

Like the Longcare parents, Norma realises she will never know exactly what happened to her son. He may have been abused. He probably was. She hopes his physical strength protected him and that Rowe tried, and failed, to abuse him. Greg doesn't talk, though, and so when Gordon Rowe died, he took his secrets with him to the grave.

'I felt so guilty, because I thought I could have done more 11 years ago,' she says. 'I felt all kinds of irrational things. People told me I wasn't guilty of anything, but I was. I will continue to blame myself for the rest of my life, because I could have done more. I am going to have to live with that and nobody is going to take that feeling of guilt away. The stark truth was... I betrayed him.'

She has tried to make up for what she sees as a failure. After Angela Rowe was released from prison, Norma wrote to the Governor of Florida, the US ambassador in London, and a police chief in Florida, warning them all that Angela might try and open a care home in the state. She also wrote to every social services director in England.

She is still furious that the complaints she made in the early 80s were not investigated more thoroughly. 'I feel badly let down by the authorities which failed miserably to minutely investigate the events in Somerset in 1982/83,' she said. She has tried unsuccessfully to find out from the London Borough of Hammersmith and Fulham, her own local authority, whether Greg's social worker ever expressed any doubts about standards of care at The Old Rectory.

For the last few years, Greg has been living very happily with a dozen or so other adults at a care home a couple of hours from London. He has his own room in the big country house and is always happy to see his mum when she comes to visit, although he never fusses when it's time for her to leave. He is taken for a twelve-fifteen mile walk every day—just a stroll for Greg—and goes shopping with staff in the nearby town. He seems happy.

Although things have improved for parents of learning disabled people since the 60s and 70s, Norma still sees young mums and dads fighting the same battles she fought more than a quarter of a century ago.

'It is slightly easier to get respite care, but they still ask—if not quite so bluntly—'why do you want respite care?' That attitude is from people who have never looked after an autistic child seven days a week, every week of the year. It is not easy. It can be very rewarding, but it is certainly not easy.'

'I think it's awful that after thirty years they are still meeting the same problems. From what I have heard from younger mums, the implication is still there that there is nothing they can do for their child, so why bother.'

39. Gary

'The government's biggest shake-up of children's services in decades, the child protection Green Paper has failed to address disabled children, according to campaigners... A national working group on child protection and disability... has called for the government to develop a national strategy to safeguard disabled children "as a matter of urgency".'

The Guardian, September 17, 2001

A few months after Angela Rowe ('voluntarily') resigned as a Longcare employee early in 1994, Gary Deacon's behaviour began to deteriorate. The allegations about abuse at the two homes had recently been published in the press and Gary's adopted father, Ron, and Doreen—Ron's second wife—were wondering what may or may not have happened to him.

Ron remembers how Gary gradually 'seemed to turn against women'. He would become upset very easily, and his angry 'tantrums' of screaming and kicking were always directed at women. 'The worst part of it was that he couldn't talk to you about what the problem was,' Ron told me.

A few weeks after the new police investigation was launched, a detective visited the Deacons. He asked some general questions about Gary and how they felt about the standard of care at Longcare, but told them at this stage there were no allegations that Gary had been abused.

Ron was one of the few who decided to leave their children at Stoke Place after the allegations were revealed in 1994. He believed Gary was better off staying with his friends, and that the standard of care had improved since Gordon and Angela Rowe left. Berkshire social services also told him there were no other vacancies near Maidenhead.

'We thought there were a few residents that were OK and Gary was one of them,' said Doreen. 'It must have been nearly a year later when Madeleine Stewart visited and told us what Angela Rowe was supposed to have done to him.'

Even now, Ron and Doreen do not know what happened to Gary at Longcare. All they have is the evidence of the brutality visited on other residents, and Lillian Lowe's statement. When Gary lost weight, staff told Ron he had been put on a diet. When his watch, new suede jacket and an electronic keyboard went missing, Ron was told they had been 'put with the good things' for safe keeping. None of these items, or scores of other presents Ron and Doreen bought for Gary, ever reappeared. It's a story familiar to nearly every Longcare parent.

Over the ten years he was at Longcare, Ron Deacon never suspected that Gary was receiving anything but the best care. 'People say to me now, 'why didn't you see anything when you were there?' But he was all right when we visited. They are not going to do anything in front of you, are they?'

'Unless there's a miracle, I know he'll be in a home for the rest of his life,' says Ron. 'Before this happened, we would have put our trust in a carer immediately, but now we think twice. We are always going to have what happened in the back of our minds, but Gary has to live somewhere.'

40. Janet

'Parents of children with severe learning disabilities in Oxfordshire are considering legal action against the county council after it moved to axe the funding of three respite care centres... The £9m cuts will include savings in services for older people (£2.5m), children and families (£2m), people with physical and learning disabilities (£3.4m) and mental health problems (£250,000).'

The Guardian, 'Society' section, April 17, 2002

Havering social services rang Pauline Hennessy to say the Bucks report had been leaked to the Press and that Gordon Rowe had been accused of raping Janet.

'At first I couldn't take it in,' she would say later. 'Not my Janet. It couldn't happen to her. I couldn't stop crying. I had always promised mum I would protect and care for Janet as if she were my own daughter. I had failed them both. How could I have let this happen? There was a tremendous feeling of guilt.'

Janet was moved from home to home in search of a permanent place to live. She moved five times in six months and put on three stone in weight. She missed her friends at Longcare and would wake up crying from nightmares.

Bit by bit, Janet began to tell Pauline what had happened to her. She said Rowe had forced her to have sex with him, that she and other members of 'Gordon's Girls' had been forced to watch pornographic videos with him, and he had slapped her around the face. She described how Gordon had videotaped 'other people' having sex with her and threatened to kill Pauline and take her children away if Janet told her what he was doing.

Pauline and her family began to realise that the signs of abuse had been there, if only they had known what to look for. The burn she 'did in cookery class'. The bruised back where she had 'slipped on the stairs', the 'sore bottom', and how Janet would say she had 'forgotten' how a certain bruise had been caused. How she would return home in shabby, torn and stained clothes, even though Pauline had bought her many bright, fashionable outfits on their frequent shopping sprees. The missing clock-radio, hair dryer, hi-fi, Walkman, television. The punishments where she was sent to her room for an hour for being rude, but which they now suspect were for days at a time. They remembered how staff had told her how Janet 'lied' and how Gordon told them not to visit so often, to 'help Janet settle in'.

'I used to phone up at 6.30pm and she was always in bed,' says Pauline. 'When she got home, she just wanted to go to bed. It never dawned on me that her medication was too high.'

Pauline remembers the way her sister would talk about Longcare after she left. 'It was fear: pure and utter fear. She told me Gordon was going to come and find her. She talked about men putting her in a van and told me her boyfriend Derek had given Gordon her new phone number.

'Later on, when she discovered Gordon had died, her emotions changed. She would sob her heart out for hours on end. She wanted to know why he had hurt her. She said he couldn't be all bad, because he said he loved her. She said, 'I didn't want Gordon to do it, I asked him to stop'. She was frightened she was going to get the blame for what he had done to her. She was so confused, because she knew that by sleeping with Gordon she had been protected from some of the other things that had been going on, some of the things he had done to her friends. I think she loved Gordon and that is why she was upset when he left, but at the same time she didn't like what he was doing to her.

'He promised her all these things to keep her sweet—a house, getting married and having children. Ever since she was a young child all she ever said was, 'I want a flat like my nan's.' She collected the estate agency adverts in the newspaper. She wanted to be normal. She wanted a boyfriend. She had three older sisters and an older brother. She saw us getting married and having a big white wedding and she wanted to get married.'

Janet often talked about the court case and told Pauline how she would tell the judge about 'the naughty people' and how he would put them in prison and all her friends would be safe. She had even chosen where all her family were to sit in court while she gave her evidence. She still talked about how one day she would get married and have a house and children of her own. But it was clear to her family that Janet no longer believed in her dreams.

On December 21, 1996, Janet died suddenly in her sleep following an epileptic seizure, a few hours after a Christmas party with other residents. She had finally found somewhere staffed with decent, well-trained people. Janet had loved her new home, but still missed her old friends from Stoke Place. Pauline believed they had finally found the permanent 'happy home' she had been seeking for her sister for so many years. The home Janet's mother, Irene, had so wanted to find before she died.

Pauline believes the stress of moving so many times, combined with the guilt and confusion of what happened to her at Longcare, were the real reasons Janet died.

'I think she just gave up,' Pauline said. 'She had been in so many different homes. In her last home, they had been giving her some counselling, which obviously pulled up a lot of memories she would rather not have thought about.'

Pauline says her relationship with her sister changed after she found out she had been abused. 'I didn't feel able to give her the comfort, because I didn't want to face the reality of the abuse. If I had the chance now, there are so many things I would do. I was so angry and all my anger was directed at Stoke Place and Buckinghamshire social services. I could deal with that, but I couldn't deal with the emotional side with Janet. If she had opened up and started talking to me, I don't know how I would have coped, because I didn't want to hear it.'

As for Gordon Rowe, she doesn't hold him as responsible for what happened as Bucks County Council. 'I think he was a pervert, but social services were there to protect these people. They were the safety net and they weren't there.' She is particularly angry that residents' families weren't informed about the incident in 1991 in which Gordon Rowe assaulted Dorothy Abbott.

'I don't think I will ever really get over what happened to Janet. She was like my daughter. I promised mum when she got her into Stoke Place that I would never forget Janet. I felt after Janet died that I had let them both down.

'For eight years I had sole responsibility for Janet. I did everything for her. The fact that she is dead now just makes it so much worse. The last three or four years of her life were such hell and I have got no way of making it better. I can't make Janet feel happy again, because she's not here.

'I miss her terribly. Every now and again I have these nightmares about the phone call; not about her dying, but about the phone call to say she had died.

'The night she died, I had spoken to her on the phone. Since she left Stoke Place, I spoke to her on the phone five or six times a day. Never once was I angry with her until that night. The children had broken up from school and there were a hundred and one things I had to do and she had already spoken to me an hour before, so I told her I didn't have time and would speak to her later. Even now, I can't believe I didn't talk to her.'

Janet's experiences at Stoke Place persuaded Pauline to set up her own home for learning disabled adults. She bought an old farmhouse in Essex and converted it into a small residential home for people with challenging behaviour. She has spent thousands of pounds training her staff, and pays them good wages. The residents' care plans are reviewed almost every week to take account of their progress. The reports from social services have been exemplary.

'Janet was in six homes in five months after she left Stoke Place,' Pauline explains. 'They were terrible and they smelt. One of them was closed down because it wasn't even registered. I thought that, eventually, once I moved off site, if Janet was still unhappy, then I would move her here. If she was ever abused or ill-treated I knew that she would have a safe place to come to.'

When she hears that some people in the care industry have told me that residential homes are better now, she replies: 'That is crap. There will always be homes and people that are bad, and I think people need to be aware of the potential for abuse, which is why I care so passionately that we must be vigilant. We are these people's only protection. Your loved ones rely on you and if you are aware of the symptoms and the possibilities and the consequences of abuse, then if unfortunately it does happen to a relative, you will know the signs to look for and where to go.

'I think every one of those members of staff that worked there, if they had tried hard enough, could have got that investigated. I say to my staff here: "If you see something you are unhappy with, bring it to my attention. If I do not deal with it, go to the inspection unit."'

41. Nicky

'The headmaster of a school for the disabled who punched and humiliated pupils was jailed for a year yesterday. Geoffrey Lloyd was reported by a woman volunteer after years of 'gratuitous violence' because teachers at Regent Special School in Tividale, West Midlands, were too scared to confront him... Lloyd from Pedmore, Stourbridge, West Midlands, admitted six charges of cruelty against three pupils.'

The Daily Telegraph, April 21, 2001

1990
Nicky Power's parents waited while the video player clicked into its routine.
A blank screen. The music starts. A jaunty Greek dance. Twanging guitars. A slow rhythm, but persistent.
The first scene: Nicky is seated at a table in a wooden chair, working at a puzzle. She squints, concentrating, behind her black frames. Then she turns and waves at the camera.
The voice begins: friendly, with a country lilt. It is the voice of

Gordon Rowe. 'This short film depicts Nicky in various stages of her progress at Stoke Place. It's not compiled in any particular order, but just shows snitbits here and there. Here, of course, she's in the classroom.'

Next to a pub, and Nicky is seated at a table, a glass of Coke in front of her, other residents nearby. She rubs the back of her head with her hand, but is too busy sucking up her drink through two straws to worry about the camera.

Soon, the video cuts to the seaside, a harbour in southern England, where Angela Rowe is untying a rope, and climbing aboard a small motor-cruiser. There are five women, including Nicky, in the boat. Nicky waves at the camera.

'Here's Angela, attending to our boat Kasba, when we took the residents on holiday to Bucklesham Bay. Our boat being moored at Chichester, we were able to give the girls who we took some very pleasant rides.'

Cut to the outbuildings in the grounds of Stoke Place. Four of the residents are gathered around a long-eared rabbit.

'Each mornin' and afternoon the residents go from the classrooms out to see the animals. Nicky loves to make close contact with them.'

Cut to the office. Nicky in a dressing-gown, her hair still wet. Staring at the camera, suddenly she smiles and waves.

'After a bath, Nicky will come down and assist me in the office. She loves me to draw houses for her, in which in the windows must be shown her grannies.'

1996

We are sitting in the Powers' conservatory, talking about their daughter, about Stoke Place. They remember watching the video and how they were reassured and impressed at how active and happy Nicky seemed under the care of Gordon Rowe.

Susan and Davyd were on holiday when news of the abuse at Longcare broke. Susan's ninety-year-old mother recognised Stoke Place in a television report. When one of the family rang Stoke Place, a member of staff told them it was 'all hearsay' and Nicky was fine.

A few days later, the Powers were visited by Nicky's social worker, from Kent County Council. He told them the truth: Nicky had been beaten and thrown and kicked down the stairs at Stoke Place. 'I was shocked,' says Susan, 'but I took it.' They decided to remove Nicky from the home. Kent social workers visited Stoke Place to talk to staff and were appalled to find there were no records for Nicky's ten years at the home, or the medication she had been given.

Just before Nicky was due to leave, the Powers received a long, rambling letter from Gordon Rowe, begging them not to take her away. He said he and Angela were planning to open a new home with small flats and they would disprove all the allegations. He said they wanted Nicky to join them at the new home, because she was one of his 'special girls'.

Within a few weeks of Nicky leaving Stoke Place, Susan and Davyd were told by their social worker that their daughter had had 'every abuse going'. They were devastated. Susan had to visit her GP for treatment for depression.

'After she moved to her new home, we were told Nicky was having up to eight baths a day and then changing her clothes,' says Susan. 'She refused to look in the mirror. She would have flashbacks and dig and scratch herself. Her key worker at the new home was just heart-broken at what had happened to her, but she has done wonders with Nicky since then.'

Susan hands over another record of Nicky's life, this one a document written several years after the boat trips and pub visits, a time when Nicky had left Stoke Place and was settling into the new home. Perhaps a more accurate record, it is a diary of Nicky's day-to-day existence as seen by the care workers helping to pick up the pieces of her life.

July 11, 1995:
Nicky spilt a cup of tea over herself in the disco. David* and Becky* took her upstairs to change. She was crying and hitting herself. David tried to stop Nicky hurting herself and in the process Nicky bent his thumb by accident. Incontinent at 2am. Perfectly OK when changed. Didn't want to wear a clean nightdress. Threw a wobbly, chewing her fist and hitting herself on the side of the head. Pacified her. Went to bed wearing a polo neck jumper.

July 12, 1995 (Nicky visits Respond, a London-based organisation that offers therapy to people with learning difficulties who have been abused):
Fine until about 2.20pm. Asked about chips (which we have on the way home). Explained we had to wait for Peter*. Started throwing books about, spitting and screaming. Trashed the waiting-room, pushed the chairs over. Kept hitting me, pulling at my clothes, ripping

my dress. After about twenty minutes, she finally calmed down and had a good cry. I gave her a cuddle. Frank* the counsellor made her a cup of tea. She then wanted to change her clothes, so Michelle* fetched her clean clothes from the car. Fine after that, laughing and looking forward to her chips.

July 14, 1995:
Nicky wanted to go up and change at 12.40pm. Took her upstairs, where she had several changes of clothes. Started getting agitated, threw one or two things and said, 'Don't do it. Don't like it.' Calmed down after a while, sat waiting for her dinner OK. On coming downstairs at 2pm, Nicky got very upset. Slapping me, Peter (very hard), screaming, spitting and generally very upset. At one stage she threw herself to the floor, dragging Barbara* down with her. Andrew* and Barbara contained her, while the staff and myself cleared the house. She then calmed down and went down to the kitchen with Lucy* and seems fine now. Blew again this afternoon in the kitchen. Christine* calmed her down, took her up to her lounge in the maisonette. Soon settled again.

5pm: Nicky wanted to change her clothes again. After supper, Nicky had soaked herself. I changed her and she blew, because she had wet herself. Wouldn't put on her clothes. Sat on her bed and wet herself again, all over me while I was changing her under garments again. Left her for a short while to calm down. Threw clothes and objects at me. Coathanger etc. Calmed down, after a while. Bathed and tried to put nightdress on. Blew again. Soaked her sheets and bedding. Changed them. At last got her into pyjamas with help from Cathy*.

July 15, 1995:
Nicky wanted to get changed at midday. Nicky asked to be changed three times this afternoon.

July 26, 1995:
Nicky was very happy and relaxed for all the journey to Wandsworth, we even had a terrible storm which she coped with very well! We arrived in good time so that they could have their packed lunch, and still Nicky was relaxed! But when Nicky's counsellor arrived, the first thing Nicky said was 'hair'. Alison then went upstairs for a short while, but on her return she asked Nicky if she was coming upstairs and that was when Nicky started her anger. She blew for a solid half an hour, hitting, spitting, but most of the problem was her spitting at Alison. We did

wonder whether anything was brought on by the fact that Alison had had her hair cut very short. All the time Nicky was angry she would look at Alison and repeat 'bye'. After Alison left we calmed her down, changed her clothes and came home, stopping for the McDonald's on the way. No more problems.

August 1, 1995:
Because Samantha* was shouting, this caused Nicky to 'blow'. We had cups, pictures flying. She then started to hit herself. After a few minutes she started to cry and then I gave her a cuddle and she slowly calmed down and went up to her room. Nicky very well behaved this evening. Bed wet, washed, changed. Quilt on the line.

Nicky was probably demonstrating the guilt and self-loathing she felt about what she had 'allowed' Gordon Rowe to do to her, and his subsequent rejection of her. Tragically, she does not realise she was not to blame.

On one visit, Susan and Nicky's care workers decided to try something different. Nicky had shown a deep hatred of all of the clothes she associated with Stoke Place—particularly the nightwear—so Susan asked her if she wanted to get rid of 'those nasty clothes'. 'Yeah, not nice,' replied Nicky. Susan took Nicky up to her bedroom and started to put the clothes in the bags. The moment she touched the clothes, Nicky flew at her, shouting, 'No, no.' It was not until they got downstairs and one of the care workers asked Nicky: 'Hi, Nick, are you going to throw those things away?' that she calmed down.

'We had to let her throw them in one of the big green bins,' says Susan. 'Then she said: "Gone," and slammed the lid down. She would not look at me. She just said: "Go." She was so frightened we were going to take her back to Stoke Place.

'Recently, I bought her a new dress and she put it on and said: "Nice, like this, I like me," and she went over to the mirror and brushed her hair. I said: "Is that all right?" and she said: "Yeah, I am nice." That was the first time she had said that for a long, long time.'

At Nicky's new home, she has her own bedroom, a pretty, comfortable place where she is surrounded by her own possessions and favourite toys. She is allowed to spend time on her own in her room at the end of the day's lessons, and is expected to help prepare meals in the small self-contained flat she shares with four other adults. Her room has its own television, and videos can be piped straight into her room if she doesn't feel like sitting downstairs with her flatmates. Quite simply, she is treated as a human being.

But Susan and Davyd were still not able to have their daughter home to visit them. She remembers their house as the place she was taken from to return to Stoke Place. Only recently would she even allow her mother to hold her hand again. Her mother was the person who always drove her back to Stoke Place.

It was only in the last few weeks that Susan Power had been able to talk about her daughter's ordeal at Stoke Place. It was August 2, 1996, nearly two years since they first read of the abuse allegations in the press, and Nicky was living in a home near London.

'The last two years have been a living hell,' Susan says, and brings out a picture of Nicky as a smiling teenager, before she moved to Stoke Place. She looked carefree and confident.

Susan produces two more snaps of her daughter, taken several years later. Nicky had started to put on weight, but the biggest change was in her eyes. The smiling confidence of her teenage years had gone, to be replaced with a haunted, ill-at-ease grimace.

For the first three or four years, Nicky seemed happy at Stoke Place. But then she began to react strangely when it was time to return to Longcare after weekend visits home. She would start to hyperventilate, and say: 'No, no, Gordon not nice, no, no, not nice.' Susan says: 'I thought she just didn't want to leave her mum and dad. When she knew we were on the M25 and heading for Stoke Place she would just shut up. We would never get another word out of her. Once or twice I brought her back after a weekend at home and I had a job to get her out of the car. I can still see her standing there, just looking so sad.'

There were other clues. 'She came home one time with a terrific bruise,' says Susan. 'All the skin on the back of her heel and her toe was crushed. I rang up Gordon and asked what on earth had happened, and he said: 'Oh, I forgot to tell you, she had a fit and fell down the stairs.' Another time I was told she had had a fit and got her foot caught under the wardrobe. On the amount of epilepsy drugs she was on, she should never have had a fit. And since she moved to her new home she hasn't had a single fit.'

They also remember Gordon Rowe's 'obsession' with Nicky's periods and how he told them he wanted all the female residents on contraceptives. They agreed, because Nicky suffered very badly with PMT.

There were other signs. Hundreds of pounds worth of gifts bought for Nicky went missing. Staff always said they were 'in the storeroom'. Rowe insisted that all money they sent to Nicky was in the form of a cheque made out to him. Again, because they trusted him, they agreed. Nicky would often come home filthy—her nails were never cut, her ears were dirty, and once there was a huge blister on one of her feet, which had been left untreated. When they arrived for a visit, they would find the residents sitting blank-eyed in front of a television screen, 'as if they had been drugged', and with no supervisor in sight. They were never encouraged to visit.

But they never considered the possibility that Nicky was being abused, either physically or sexually. 'I never thought about it,' says Susan. 'I suppose we just trust people. Because you would never do it, you don't think other people would.'

Davyd Power remembers Christmases, when Nicky would come home with armfuls of gifts from Gordon. 'Whether it was conscience money, I don't know, but he always said Nicky was one of his favourites.'

It was eighteen months later. I was sitting again in the Powers' home in Tonbridge. We were talking about the slow improvements Nicky had made since we last met. They were still worried about the heavy doses of anti-epilepsy drugs she had to take—her doctor was apprehensive about weaning her off them after so long. Nicky was gradually losing weight, she changed her clothes less regularly, but still couldn't stand people coming upstairs or downstairs behind her. Her parents didn't know how long she would continue to receive counselling from Respond, but it appeared to be working, slowly. She even seemed to be getting her sense of humour back and now had a boyfriend, who proudly told Susan and Davyd on a recent visit that he had just made their daughter breakfast—Nicky covered her face with her hands.

Despite her progress, Nicky had almost had a 'breakdown' the previous year. She wrecked one of the rooms at Respond during a counselling session. One moment she was totally withdrawn and uncommunicative, the next frenziedly ripping at her dress, scratching, pinching and punching herself and those around her. Alison, the counsellor, wouldn't tell them the content of the sessions. They were confidential, between her and Nicky, she said. For a few months, the counselling had to stop, but it had now started again.

*

Early December 1999, more than five years since Longcare first made headlines, and Nicky still shows no signs of forgetting. She still has nightmares. She will throw her pine bedroom furniture across the room, shouting and smashing the drawers and turning on the taps to try to flood the room. She pulls out clumps of her hair and claws herself. These rages often occur on Saturday afternoons, after she has had a counselling session in the morning. And while she is raging, she will repeat the words: 'Gordon not nice, don't do it.'

The Powers realise Nicky will never forget what happened to her at Longcare, and they will never know even half of what she went through. She is scarred for life. Now Susan just wants to know what happened to her daughter at Stoke Place. 'Then if anything happens later on—if she "turns" again—we could look back and say: "That's why."'

For a while, Nicky lost her love of animals. A visit to an animal sanctuary with other residents brought back disturbing memories and, in her mother's words, 'all hell let loose'. But on a recent walk in the forest with her parents, Nicky was able to stroke one of the horses. She can also now visit the pub, enjoy hydrotherapy sessions at the swimming pool and occasionally take part in the dinner parties the residents help their care workers organise every three weeks. Sometimes her care workers take her out for a meal—she likes Indian and Chinese food—and her table manners are improving again. And she still loves her Abba tapes.

Nicky's latest care plan shows some improvement. She will go on outings, but still has a problem with people touching her hair. Her periods of 'being distressed' vary from once a day to six or seven times a day, and sometimes she gets through a day without any outbursts. After an episode she will be 'very nice' to staff and apologise. She has also hit out at other residents.

She is calmer than when she arrived at the home. She only wets herself once or twice a week, rather than 'all day, every day', but still has severe depression. Susan doesn't believe Nicky will ever come to terms with what happened to her at Stoke Place. 'I think she blames us deep down because I expect she feels that when she said, 'Gordon, not nice', she was trying to tell us in her own way, and we didn't know and we kept taking her back.

'I try to trust them at her new home because they were all so horrified at what happened to her and because of the way they have worked with her.'

This year, her parents are hoping to bring her home for Christmas Day for the first time for five years, although it will depend on how she is feeling on the day. Visits still only last about forty minutes, before Nicky will say: 'Where's Helen* [one of the care assistants]? Go see Helen now.' She is happy to see her parents go and waves goodbye from the window.

Susan Power believes that what happened at Stoke Place shows how society treats learning disabled people as second-class citizens.

'You can see a lot of disgust on people's faces, they tend to pull their children away. When she was younger and was screaming and screaming I used to get people saying: "That child needs a damn good wallop," or "that mother's got no control over her daughter".' 'Quite a lot of people still think they should be put away and not seen.'

42. Simon

> 'Because he has Down's syndrome and is mentally handicapped the doctor asked us if we wanted to leave him to slowly slip away.'
>
> From the mother of a seven-year-old child with heart problems. Extract from a report on discrimination in the NHS against people with Down's Syndrome: Down's Syndrome Association, March 1999

Avril and Brian Scott didn't know anything about the allegations against Rowe until August, 1994, when they received a call from Simon's social worker. She told them she wanted to take Simon away from Stoke Place, but couldn't tell them why. The Scotts drove immediately to Stoke Poges and spoke to Ray Cradock. He told them Bucks County Council was trying to 'stitch up' Gordon Rowe because it owed him money. The truth will all come out in the end, he said, and told them to take no notice of the 'rumours'. Although the Scotts didn't trust Ray Cradock, they decided to let Simon stay at Stoke Place, because they believed he was happy there.

A few weeks later, Avril and Brian received another call from their social worker. She told them there had been an investigation at Longcare and it was far more serious than the story Ray Cradock had spun them. The county council's report mentioned that Simon had been denied treatment for his epilepsy, because staff thought he was faking his symptoms. This time, the Scotts drove down to Stoke Place and brought Simon home. The result was a call from Ray Cradock, who wrongly accused them of making threatening phone calls.

Avril and Brian Scott tell me they were generally 'very happy' with Longcare, although the attitude of some of the staff and 'one or two other little things' disturbed them. Once, Simon told them how a care assistant smacked his bottom; another time, that he was sent to his room because he had been naughty. He also told them about Jackie being dragged out of the dining-room because she wouldn't eat her dinner. But they didn't worry; they believed Gordon Rowe had a 'soft spot' for their son—he used to call him 'Randolph' (after the actor, Randolph Scott), and was always laughing and joking with him when they visited. Brian and Gordon often discussed their mutual interest in videos and filming, and Rowe once showed him his impressive studio in the cottage.

But, sometimes, Simon would return home for the weekend and they wouldn't be able to get a word out of him—they now believe it was because of the regime of drugs Gordon Rowe had placed him on. Avril tells me Simon was 'one of the lucky ones', because they phoned him so often and Gordon and her husband were so friendly.

Brian says Simon was better off at Stoke Place—he was fitter, because of all the exercise he received working in the grounds as one of the 'working lads', and he seemed to 'thrive' on the harsh regime. But Avril disagrees. Simon has put on weight since leaving Stoke Place and is much happier. 'He's so much more content, it's incredible,' she tells me. 'He doesn't stop talking now—we even have to tell him to be quiet sometimes. He phones us up every night.'

When I meet Simon, his memories of Stoke Place are vague and distant. It is 1998 and Simon is well settled into a 'lovely' home in Essex, living 'semi-independently' in a flat with an autistic friend, and is gradually returning to the young man his parents used to know. Both of them are former Longcare residents. His friend's only communication about his time at the home has been to draw a picture of Stoke Place, with bombs falling on it from the sky.

Simon remembers the 'big old building' and how he would feed the animals and work in the gardens every day. But he also recalls his friend Fred being locked in his room because he 'lost his temper'. And he remembers Gordon Rowe. 'He said you must not do that. He told me off. He taught me to drink beer,' he tells me. Gordon, he says, called him and his friend 'the terrible twins'.

But Avril remembers the hints of a darker side to Simon's time at Stoke Place. 'Twice he was made to stand outside, because he had dirty shoes on, and he was made to take all his clothes off. Somebody kicked him up the bottom. We visited him one time and there was one lad with Down's syndrome who was being made to stand behind one of the pillars until he was called, and I remember Simon saying: 'Uh-oh, he's been naughty.'

'Every time we went up there, Simon had stitches in his forehead or on his nose or had a burn on his arm. There were so many little niggly things that you accepted at the time, but now it's all come out you realise...' She pauses. 'There was another time when we were all together in the car and Simon said to me, completely out of the blue: 'I do not put my fits on'.' She hesitates again. 'He was one of the lucky ones, because we phoned up every week,' she says finally. But it is clear she doesn't entirely believe what she is saying.

It isn't just Simon who has to recover from Longcare. 'We are still trying to get over what happened, because we feel guilty,' Avril tells me. 'It was our decision to send him there. Why didn't we see the signs? All the parents feel the same way, but it doesn't help the guilt. It is our fault that he went through what he did.'

Every now and again, something happens to Simon to trigger a memory. Avril remembers receiving a phone call from her son several months before. He was upset. A member of staff had told him he would be sent away if he didn't make his bed. When Avril phoned the home, she discovered it was something Simon had remembered being told at Stoke Place.

When I speak to them three years later, the Scotts are still finding it difficult to trust anyone who cares for their son, despite the excellent care he now receives.

Life hasn't been easy for Simon in the last three years, even if his memories of Longcare appear to be fading. In August 1998, he had a severe seizure. One of the care assistants called an ambulance. While they were waiting, his heart stopped. The care assistant managed to resuscitate him, but he spent the next 12 days in intensive care. His kidneys also failed and Simon spent four weeks receiving dialysis. Fortunately, he made a full recovery. 'We nearly lost him,' says Avril.

'It took him a long time to get over it,' adds Brian. 'We virtually had to teach him to walk again.'

When he returned to Essex, he was moved to a flat on the ground floor. 'He's had his ups and downs,' says Brian. 'On the floor he is on at the moment, there are wheelchair people who are physically but not mentally impaired and they have not got any patience with him. There is nothing too bad, but the staff did suggest a move. They are going to move him to an upstairs room now that he has settled down, where he will be with people he can communicate with. There is one friend he has with Down's syndrome. They get on really well and Simon is always popping up to see him or he's coming down to see Simon.'

Simon can dress, toilet and feed himself, and operate the video, television and music centre his parents have bought him. But he could never live on his own. He's happy where he is. 'He loves it,' says Avril. 'It's his home.' Despite this measure of independence, he still calls his parents every evening. 'He's been on the phone tonight,' Brian tells me. 'He goes to college on Mondays and they have stopped doing dinners. They have now got to take a packed lunch and he reckons he can take whatever he wants. He's going to let me know on Saturday what he wants to take.'

Simon still comes home every weekend to see his parents and whenever his favourite programme, 'Who Wants To Be A Millionaire' starts on television, Simon immediately rings up his dad to tell him to switch it on. 'He tells me to phone up the number to get on it so I can win lots of money for him,' says Brian.

Brian no longer believes that Simon escaped punishment at Longcare. But he thinks his son managed to keep in favour with Rowe, and probably escaped the worst of the abuse. 'I think he knew that if he did what he was told, he kept out of trouble. He was a little bit apprehensive of the Rowes, so he would toe the line.'

In the years following his departure from Stoke Place, Simon would occasionally mention the home and Gordon Rowe. But in the last couple of years he has stopped talking about Longcare. 'He never mentions it at all,' says Brian. 'A couple of times we have given him an opening when he could, but he hasn't.'

'Bits came out every now and again, but not now. I think he's closed that off in his brain now,' says Avril.

Even though Simon may be getting over his experiences, Avril says, 'We don't trust anybody. It's terrible to say it, but that's what it comes down to in the end. Question everything. Every time they phone up and say he's not very well and can't come to the phone, we question it. Every time he comes home with a bruise, we question it. We have to question everything. It's the only way, because if there is one thing we have learned from this, it is that you can't trust anybody, because people like Simon are so vulnerable.'

43. Stefano

> 'In 1999, 13.7 per cent of all residential staff in Wales had a formal qualification.'
>
> Social Services Inspectorate for Wales: Social Services in Wales 1999-2000—*The Report of the Chief Inspector*, January 2001

It was only after Desmond Tully left Stoke Place in 1990 that the Tunstells began to have regular contact with Gordon Rowe. But as he became 'more prominent' in Stefano's care, they became steadily more concerned about what care at the home and at the high doses of tranquillisers their son was given.

'I told the social worker that I must take him away from there,' says Lidia. 'She asked for time to talk to everybody in her team. I kept putting pressure on and we had him home every weekend.

'At the end of January, 1993, we had a phone call from a new social worker and he said to us, "I think it's not safe for Stefano to stay there." He never really said why, but he said he felt that Stefano had been abused. We took him home.'

The police investigation launched in September, 1994, uncovered a series of allegations that Stefano had been ill-treated. They began in 1987, with an incident in which he was said to have been sitting on a chair with a dish of pudding on his lap, shovelling the food into his mouth. Desmond Tully allegedly hit him on the chin and took him out of the room. Tully was later cleared of this charge during the trial at Kingston Crown Court.

On another occasion, a member of staff saw Stefano holding his head and shouting: 'No! No!' at Gordon Rowe. One care assistant saw Rowe holding Stefano by his shoulders on a toilet as he tried to get up. Another described Rowe filling a beaker of cold water and pouring it over him: there was no reaction from Stefano.

Towards the end of his stay, after Stefano wet himself in one of the classrooms, Rowe accused him of doing it deliberately and told staff that he should stand outside in his wet clothes until he was dry. If he wet himself at mealtimes, Stefano had to eat his meals outside, no matter how cold it was or whether it was raining. Witnesses saw Rowe drag Stefano outside by his ears and clothes.

Following an unsuccessful couple of years at a residential home near Hastings, Stefano was found a place at a home closer to London.

He gradually settled in. The quantities of drugs he takes have been drastically reduced, but, now in his early thirties, he is still 'up and down' and 'not really himself'. His parents wonder whether he will ever return to the happy and sensitive young man they knew before he moved to Stoke Place, the young man who enjoyed going for walks and listening to classical music.

'I feel as though sometimes he doesn't trust anyone, that he's giving up,' says Lidia. 'He is quite depressed and I never know how he will be the next time we see him. He has such a terrible disability to cope with and what happened to him—how can he get over it? He needs some sort of help.' The agency that looks after him decided he would not benefit from counselling, but recommended music and art therapy.

Stefano's incontinence has improved, but the Tunstells have been told by the home's owner, a psychologist, that he was almost certainly sexually abused.

'I know he suffered a lot,' says Lidia. 'It's difficult to know exactly what happened to him there, but there were bits and pieces that happened when he returned home that probably came from his past. He had this habit of pulling us from armchairs when we were sitting down—we just don't know what happened to him there to make him do this. He would also make these strange noises. These were things he never did before Stoke Place.

'He is better now, but I don't think he will ever recover. He was a very happy boy before he went to Stoke Place. Now he hardly ever smiles and he will push us away. He prefers to be on his own now. This is his way of expressing his frustration and the anger he feels that we allowed this to happen, as if it is our own fault.

'We put our extremely vulnerable child in a home, not because we wanted to get rid of him but because we thought maybe they could help him and he would mix with other people. But they abused him in every sense. I don't trust anyone after that place, wherever he goes. I can never relax. When he's not here, I always worry about him. Before he went there, the possibility of abuse never crossed my mind. I can't believe that such a thing could happen to a person with so many problems.'

Lidia wishes Rowe was still alive so that he could be punished for his crimes. But he is not the main focus of her anger.

'Gordon Rowe took the money and he treated these people like animals—worse than animals. But to be honest I feel more angry with Buckinghamshire social services. They knew about his record, they knew he had done something wrong. How could this man have had such a job with such vulnerable people?'

Now she only wants to know what happened to Stefano at Stoke Place. Amazingly, she had no idea Desmond Tully had been tried in court for allegedly punching her son, until I told her nearly twelve months after Tully was cleared of the charge.

'I really want to know what happened,' she told me. 'I don't think I can really be at peace until I know who was responsible for what happened to him.'

Lidia believes that what happened at Longcare proved the need for more frequent and thorough inspections of care homes, paying more attention to how the residents feel about the care they are receiving.

But she says the main problem is the attitude of the public towards people with learning difficulties. 'They are second class citizens. I try not to tell people I have an autistic child. Often when I say he is autistic there is a big, big silence. If I say he is in a home they say that it is their taxes that are paying for children like ours. They say, 'You're lucky not to have to look after him at home.' That's all I get, so usually I don't say anything. There isn't a great deal of sympathy for people like Stefano. We had people say to us: 'Well, being so handicapped, he would never have understood what was happening to him.' But he's a human being and he's very sensitive.

'Logically, I know I didn't have any choice in doing what I did, but as a mother I always have this feeling of failure. I feel that perhaps when I saw the first signs I should have just picked him up and taken him home, but you know that if he loses sponsorship from the local authority it is very difficult to get it back. You have to follow the system. I felt I couldn't possibly manage to look after him all day. That's the situation, but it doesn't make me feel any better.'

Lidia has been taking anti-depressants to help her cope with the feelings of guilt and failure. The abuse Stefano was subjected to has wrecked her life, just as it wrecked his. 'I hide myself in my job, but when I am on my own, especially at the weekend, everything comes back to me. I don't like to go anywhere. It's only my job that makes me go out,' she says.

She and her husband worry about what will happen to Stefano when they are dead. 'We are getting older and I have been very ill. We will not be here for ever. Who is going to keep an eye on him? Nobody. I can't trust anybody. What if something happened again? It could happen.'

44. Justice for Longcare Survivors

> 'Since joining, my life has changed so much. I've met so many interesting people, it is really rewarding. Now I have the confidence to speak up for myself. It's so different, the people here actually listen to me. I now feel like a complete person, it's given me so much confidence to believe in myself. Everyone here has made me feel so welcome. I no longer feel like I'm a label or a hassle to anyone. We all work together here and I really enjoy being part of a team.'
>
> Member of Skills for People, an organisation based in Newcastle upon Tyne, which supports people with physical and/or learning difficulties to speak up for themselves

The name of Rowe's creation was to live on. In the months following the first reports about Longcare, relatives of the victims began to make contact with each other. They linked up through the charities which made public pronouncements, such as Voice UK and Mencap, through contacts they had made during visits to the homes in years gone by, and through acquaintances made at the Longcare trial.

Although a tiny handful of relatives maintained unwavering loyalty towards Longcare, most were heartbroken by what had happened, and were relieved that there were others in similar positions they could go to for support.

Two of the most active and outspoken relatives were Pauline Hennessey and June Raybaud, Janet Ward's sister and aunt. They proved to be strong and determined campaigners, both by becoming trustees of the charity Voice UK, which helps learning disabled people who have experienced crime or abuse, and by launching and co-ordinating the new support group for Rowe's victims.

The group decided on a name: Justice for Longcare Survivors. Together, its members began their long journey towards an acknowledgement that what had been done to their loved ones was wrong. But they also wanted the government to recognise the flaws in the system that had helped Rowe commit his crimes and get away with them for so long, and to put them right.

At the first meeting in 1996, a room full of thirty or so relatives had discussed their memories of Longcare.

One man stood up to say that his son's television had gone missing while he was at Stoke Place: Rowe told him it was being mended, and he never saw it again. Other relatives stood up and told their stories: the unexplained bruises, the over-medication.

It was a frustratingly slow process, but at least those who attended JLS meetings knew they were doing something, not only to make things better for their loved ones, but to push for improvements that might prevent another Longcare.

By late 2000, the members of JLS had been meeting regularly for nearly four years, maintaining a careful catalogue of their and the victims' recollections of Longcare.

Probably their most important victory had been to ensure that the findings of the Independent Longcare Inquiry were published. They had also shamed five senior officers from Bucks County Council into attending one of their meetings. The grudging apology for the inspection unit's mistakes that resulted from that meeting did not go far enough, but it was something.

The members of JLS had also decided to take legal action against the people they blamed for what happened at Longcare. After all, their sons and daughters were going to need specialist care in the years ahead to cope with the after-effects of the abuse, so why shouldn't the organisations responsible help pay for this care. Apart from anything, such compensation would be a recognition that what had been done was wrong. It would act as a warning shot across the bows of other inspection authorities, police forces, and care homes.

They were eventually told that they would not be able to sue the Rowes, Lorraine Field or Desmond Tully, because the Legal Services

Commission did not believe they had enough money to make it worth their while to fund the cases. In response, the JLS group asked their lawyers to track down Angela and Nigel Rowe and find out what had happened to Gordon Rowe's millionaire's playthings—the holiday home, the boat, the sports car. They also decided to look into Desmond Tully's financial background as he too had previously owned his own residential home in Devon, now run by a relative, and it was rumoured that he owned other properties. The two solicitors who represented most of the Longcare victims, Nicola Harney, of Stewarts, in London, and Simon Richardson, of The Smith Partnership, in Derby, employed a private detective to make some preliminary investigations in Florida, but the search would ultimately prove fruitless.

JLS and their lawyers had reluctantly decided not to sue any of the local authorities that placed clients at Longcare, or Thames Valley Police, and instead to concentrate on Buckinghamshire County Council. Despite the suspicion that many of those placing authorities had abandoned their clients at the homes, it was felt they could provide useful information for the case against Bucks. Legal precedent suggested a claim against the police would not succeed. They, too, were considered a good source of evidence. Again, it was a decision many relatives found hard to accept.

As the months and years passed, the numbers who attended the meetings dwindled. But there was always a solid core of parents, many of whom had retired, or were self-employed and found it easier to spare the time. Stefano Tunstell's parents, Lidia and Leslie, often attended; June and Pauline; Shaun McCarthy's parents, Terry and Barbara, who made it to nearly every meeting until they moved to Devon in 2000; Avril and Brian Scott; Rose Terry, whose sister Linda Dagger was a Longcare resident, and her husband Bill; Benedict Alcindor, Rosie's aunt; and Olive and Ken Everitt, whose daughter Tracy was at Longcare. Many others came a couple of times a year to keep up-to-date.

These get-togethers helped convince the families they were making progress, kept them in contact with sympathetic friends, and, most importantly, proved they were doing something to make up for that one tragic mistake they had all made: trusting Gordon Rowe.

The regular JLS meetings also helped the compilation of evidence necessary for the civil case against Buckinghamshire County Council.

In 2003, a trial date was finally set: October 13, at the Royal Courts of Justice in London. The trial judge had ruled that he would hear only the details of Janet Ward's case. If that case was proved, all the other claimants against Bucks would also succeed.

45. An Affront to Human Dignity

> 'When Mabel first came to the group, she didn't speak at all, because in St Lawrence's, if you said anything, they said, 'shut up!'. Now she has written her life story, she has been on TV, she has been all round Europe setting up People First groups. That is someone who would not say anything but 'yes' and 'no'. Now she would stand up against anybody. The tragedy is to think of the potential she had.'
>
> Kathy Thompson, social worker and People First supporter, discussing People First member Mabel Cooper, a former patient of St Lawrence's long-stay hospital

It had been obvious from the first months of working on the Longcare story that there were many flaws in the social care and criminal justice systems that exposed learning disabled people to abuse. But, as the years passed, was anything being done to correct them?

Six years on from Bucks County Council's Longcare probe, many inspection units were still proving themselves incapable of exposing abuse. This was one of the main reasons for the introduction of the Care Standards Act 2000.

Many of its measures were strongly influenced by the conclusions of Tom Burgner's Longcare report. One of the most important was to set up a National Care Standards Commission (NCSC), which would replace inspection units, and assume responsibility for registration and inspection of about 35,000 care homes, domiciliary care agencies and children's homes in England, and make sure they met tough new standards. Similar bodies were launched in Wales and Scotland. The commission was supposed to be independent, immune from the politics and constant funding crises of local government and would offer consistent registrations and inspections across the country. Most importantly, perhaps, it pledged that its inspectors would spend more time talking to the residents/service-users during their visits.

But less than three weeks after the commission was launched in April, 2002, the government announced that it would be abolished within two years, and its social care functions merged with the Social Services Inspectorate to form a new Commission for Social Care Inspection. It was a signal for further confusion to come.

The Care Standards Act also set up a General Social Care Council. The council, with equivalent bodies in Northern Ireland, Wales and Scotland, would regulate the estimated 1.5 million staff in England's care industry. It would gradually set up a social care register of all those seen as fit to be working in the sector, and regulate training and education. Amazingly, it was the first time there had ever been a regulatory organisation for the social care industry. There was also to be a new list of people considered unfit to be working with vulnerable adults: the Protection of Vulnerable Adults (POVA) list. This would give learning disabled people the same protection the Protection of Children Act list gave children. An employer would be obliged to notify the government if she dismissed a member of staff for harming or risking harm to a client.

At long last a potentially effective measure was to be introduced. Except, it was never implemented. Thanks to the chaos generated by problems at the newly privatised Criminal Records Bureau (CRB), the government announced in the autumn of 2002 that the introduction of POVA had been indefinitely deferred.

But the Care Standards Act also said that all staff working in care homes would have to undergo criminal records checks by the end of March 2003. Thanks to the CRB chaos, this deadline was extended to the end of 2004. Furthermore, the government announced that plans to force all staff working for domiciliary care agencies to have CRB checks were also being suspended. Care workers who wanted to work with vulnerable adults would merely have to sign a statement saying that they had no criminal convictions—in other words they would be asked to complete their own (privatised) CRB checks.

But that wasn't all, either. The General Social Care Council admitted to me that it could take ten years before all care workers were admitted onto its new social care register, the launch of which was already being delayed by the CRB fiasco.

This was all taking place only weeks after the government had announced, following months of concerted lobbying by care home owners, that existing homes would not, after all, have to meet many of the new standards relating to physical layout and facilities. As Anne Parker, chair of the NCSC, said: 'The hard core of providers, who've let the sector down over many years by delivering poor standards to their residents, may take comfort, sit back, and then do nothing to bring their facilities up to a decent standard.'

Telling was an admission from then Home Office minister Lord Falconer that measures relating to staff working with vulnerable adults were being postponed, while those concerning staff working with children were not, because the safety of children was a higher priority than learning disabled people.

Potentially good legislation had been backsliding fast as a result of underfunding. And, as usual when it came to priorities, learning disabled people were at the bottom of the pile.

Then, in March 2001, the Government published *Valuing People*, the first White Paper on learning disability since *Better Services for the Mentally Handicapped* in 1971. It was greeted with some applause by many voluntary organisations. *Community Care* magazine described it as a 'defining moment'. The White Paper talked at length about the importance of civil rights, independence, choice and inclusion for people with learning difficulties.

There was to be a national information centre and help-line for care workers, in partnership with Mencap, and the development of a national network of advocacy services. The White Paper also set targets for improving access and combating discrimination in health, housing, education, social security, public transport and employment.

There would be guidance from the Department of Health on the use of restraint techniques by care workers, and a new training framework that hopefully would increase the proportion of trained staff in residential care. And there was a string of other targets, taskforces, support teams and partnership boards. The White Paper placed a refreshing emphasis on the rights of learning disabled people to make decisions for themselves and to achieve independence.

But where was the money? The White Paper said there would be £100 million over two years for a learning disability development fund—much of which would be diverted from pre-existing funding—an implementation support fund of £2.3 million a year and a £2 million learning disability research programme.

The annual spending on services for people with learning difficulties was about £3 billion, roughly split between health and social services. An extra £30 million a year new money did not add enough.

The charity Mencap said in January, 2003, that the government 'had made no attempt to assess how much it will cost to implement *Valuing People* and do not see it as a priority'. It estimated that the government would need to spend £300 million on services to achieve the vision set out in *Valuing People*.

Rob Greig, director of implementation for *Valuing People*, told me that his £2 million-odd a year budget 'patently isn't a lot of money'. 'It limits what we can do. It means we have to very carefully prioritise what we work on,' he said.

If there was one problem area on which the different groups generally agreed, it was the question of low paid care staff. Care home standards are unlikely to rise until staff wages and training improved dramatically. At the end of 2000, up to four fifths of residential care staff in England and Wales were untrained. Many of the rest had unsuitable qualifications.

In 2002, a Joseph Rowntree Foundation report[1] stated: 'In one of the more affluent areas studied, people could earn more than £10 per hour for working behind a bar, compared with an average £5 an hour for care work.'

Residential care work is rarely seen as a career. Care home owners fail to invest, or cannot afford to invest, in training. Central government and local authorities do not provide the money to fund the higher fees that might allow owners to pay higher wages. The result is an unmotivated and poorly trained workforce. That means poor standards of care and a heightened risk of ill-treatment and abuse.

As Nick Johnson, assistant chief executive of the Social Care Association, said: 'If you valued people, you would not let untrained people near [people with learning difficulties].'

This concern about the quality and quantity of care workers was shared by Clare Johnson, one of the Longcare whistle-blowers. Seven years after leaving Longcare, and by now an experienced care worker, she was appalled at the attitudes and skills of many of those working in the care system. There were some genuine care workers, she told me, but many others were either bullies seeking power over vulnerable people, or low-skilled workers who couldn't find employment anywhere else and were terrified of losing their jobs.

There are recruitment problems in local government, too. The number of people applying to be social workers has fallen sharply, with many local authorities increasingly struggling to fill posts. Many social service departments, especially those in London and the south-east, are forced to rely heavily on agency staff or recruit from aboard. The bad press suffered by social workers over the last ten years has had a drastic knock-on effect on the numbers of young people wanting to enter the profession. Although the government has responded with a recruitment drive in October 2001, there is no sign of an end to the crisis.

Despite the various government-inspired mistakes, there is no doubt that the principles behind the NCSC were good. For one thing, the commission might encourage people like Clare Johnson to come forward and report abuse. Many of the Longcare staff—even those experienced in residential care—did not know who to make allegations to. As a young and inexperienced care assistant, Clare had felt frightened, intimidated and powerless, until she was given the inspection unit's number by a colleague and told they wanted to speak to her.

But it is even more important that learning disabled people themselves know how to complain. The charity Respond is trying to address this problem. When it updated its website in 2002, it provided easy-to-follow advice, pictures describing what abuse is and details on how victims can contact Respond for further advice. The site is aimed at the increasing numbers of learning disabled people who have access to the internet. At present, it is only an option for those with milder learning difficulties. But, in the future, with continued technological advances, it may be possible even for more severely disabled people to take advantage of such a service, and learn to report abuse by themselves.

One of the major failures in the system highlighted by the Longcare case was the inability of different agencies to work together, in particular the police, social services and health authorities. Hopefully, the NCSC, and its successor, the Commission for Social Care Inspection, will become as widely known in the industry as Ofsted is among teachers, which could only help to show care workers the right people to talk to. If all the official bodies that had had contact with the Longcare residents had pooled and compared their information, the abuse would have been brought to a halt many years earlier than it was.

In the spring of 2000, the government further tried to address this by issuing *No Secrets*, guidance on how local authorities should develop their own 'multi-agency' codes of practice to help protect vulnerable adults from abuse. Each social services department, together with all other relevant agencies, such as the police and health authorities, had to implement the framework by October 2001. The aim of the guidance, which referred to the Longcare case, was both to make protection and the investigation of allegations of abuse more co-ordinated and coherent.

Although, by late 2002, it appeared that most local authorities had produced their own adult protection policies, *No Secrets* had not been allocated sufficient money for implementation. According to research[2], few councils had specific budgets for adult protection and many of those expected those budgets to disappear in the future. Furthermore, the government was showing no interest in monitoring local authorities' performance on adult protection, as it did with child protection.

Once again, the government had betrayed its true colours: protecting learning disabled people was not, and never would be, a priority.

The word priority has always been a useful one in analysing the government's actions to help people with learning difficulties. Chancellor Gordon Brown made it quite clear where he thought the priorities lay when he announced the results of his Comprehensive Spending Review in July 2002. Even though he announced that social services spending as a whole would rise by 29 per cent by 2004, there would be no new money for learning disability. Rob Greig told me he had been 'disappointed' with the decision.

He should not have been surprised. As Alan Corbett, of Respond, told me: 'The battle to get funding for therapy for people who have been sexually abused seems to be getting worse. There is a real lack of money there for the treatment that they really need. All the work that has gone on to ensure that people are valued more seems to stand for nothing when we actually get down to seeing what the national priorities are.'

It was a view shared by Brian White, co-chairperson of the government's National Forum of People with Learning Difficulties. He wrote in *Community Care* in November 2002: 'People with Learning Difficulties have never been a priority... I think that in years to come we will see right through the selfishness of governments that have never given us a second thought. They only do something when it is beneficial to them, and if it's not, they don't bother.'

David Behan, the new president of the Association of Directors of Social Services, told the same magazine his five priorities for the next year. Children were on the list, so were older people. But there was no sign of people with learning difficulties.

The government's new health and social care priorities, also announced in the autumn of 2002, did not include people with learning difficulties, even though they are the most discriminated against, poorest, most vulnerable sector of society—the focus was on children, older people and those with mental health problems.

Furthermore, the Department of Health admitted to me that it had no plans to fund any research aimed at discovering how prevalent the abuse of people with learning difficulties actually was.

Valuing People came thirty years after its predecessor. That, too, had talked about collaboration between health and social services, and providing co-ordinated advice and practical help for care workers. That White Paper had also talked about phasing out the use of long-stay hospitals for residential care and the importance of staff training. It had also talked about the vital role played by friends, neighbours and voluntary groups. And it, too, had failed to come up with the money to bring about those changes.

The legal system was one of the most vital areas for reform thrown up by the Longcare case. In some ways, it was *the* most vital. Gordon Rowe knew how difficult it was to bring a successful prosecution for crimes committed against a person with a learning difficulty, particularly for sexual offences. There was little risk of arrest, and even less of conviction.

It was obvious that magistrates, solicitors, barristers, and especially judges and Crown Prosecution Service staff urgently needed to be taught how to deal sensitively and intelligently with learning disabled people who entered the criminal justice system.

Unfortunately, the judiciary is a crusty and irritable beast, and doesn't take kindly to advice from outsiders. It has refused to undertake specific training on learning difficulty issues, although new guidelines on people with disabilities have been issued to all judges as part of the Judicial Studies Board's equal treatment bench book. The book does include some helpful points. For instance, it offers advice on reducing the stress felt by vulnerable witnesses and on how to take their evidence. But judges need to go further than that. They need specific training, and must be forced to put that training into practice.

Fiona Mactaggart told the Commons in February 2002: 'I have spoken to the chair of the Judicial Studies Training Board, who is proud of the fact that judges receive half a day's training on disability. If they receive half a day's training on disability, how much training do they receive in learning disability and ways of communicating with people with learning disabilities? It is not enough. Until we introduce serious training on how to communicate with people with learning disabilities for police, prosecutors and judges, we shall fail to deliver justice.'

This was confirmed by *Disability Now*, which reported in November 2002 how new research[3] showed judges were failing to help witnesses with learning difficulties give their best evidence in court. The researchers found that judges rarely intervened to stop prosecuting barristers harassing learning disabled witnesses or asking them confusing questions.

Perhaps the biggest obstacle to justice, though, has been the attitude of the Crown Prosecution Service. Too many cases have fallen by the wayside, because the CPS decided there was no realistic chance of successful prosecutions where the victim and main witness had a learning difficulty. Sometimes, this reluctance has been justified. The courts are, after all, heavily tilted against learning disabled people. But it was clear the CPS lacked the specialist knowledge to deal with cases where the victim and/or witness had a learning difficulty. Often, this went further than a mere absence of knowledge, and reached as far as ignorance, discrimination and prejudice.

Many crown prosecutors seemed to dismiss the idea of learning disabled people appearing as potential witnesses, without even meeting them. Many other cases reached the courts, often because a determined police officer had pushed for a prosecution, only for the CPS to pull out before the case reached trial.

By the end of 2002, there was at least a commitment among CPS bosses to try to improve the way it dealt with cases involving people with learning difficulties. The Ann Craft Trust, a learning disability charity, had been awarded the contract to train CPS staff. Ann Craft director Deborah Kitson told me she believed there was a 'real commitment' within the CPS to improve, with every lawyer now to receive three days training on learning disability.

The following year, in September 2003, the CPS and the charity Voice UK organised a conference aimed at improving communication between prosecutors and learning disabled people. Sir David Calvert-Smith QC, director of public prosecutions, said the CPS was doing 'considerable amounts of training'. The conference heard details of a Merseyside scheme that had supported learning disabled witnesses to give evidence in a series of 20 trials which followed a massive police investigation into abuse in residential homes in the north-west.

But the conference heard there were persistent problems in other parts of the country, where police officers and crown prosecutors continued to write off learning disabled victims as undependable witnesses who 'tell lies' and 'change their stories'.

Inevitably, efforts to improve the system were being hampered by funding problems. One prosecutor told the conference: 'We need more support staff to offer those services and the money just isn't there to do that.'

There were plenty of other barriers within the criminal justice system. Chief among them was the way learning disabled people were treated in the court-room itself. Historically, little attention had been paid to making it easier for such witnesses to give evidence.

Parts of the Youth Justice and Criminal Evidence Act 1999 were intended to put that right. One of the most important parts of the act stated that learning disabled people would now be assumed to be competent to appear on the witness stand, rather than assumed to be incompetent, as was previously the case. The act would also allow witnesses to give evidence unsworn, if they found it difficult to understand the oath.

There was a range of other measures which would, in theory, help more people with learning difficulties give evidence. Under the act, those acting for a witness with a learning difficulty could ask the judge for various 'special measures'. These include the use of screens to prevent intimidation by the accused in the dock; the removal of wigs and gowns by court officials; and the use of video-links, allowing a vulnerable witness to give evidence outside the court-room. Although the act became law in 1999, these measures were only due to be introduced in crown courts from August, 2002, thirteen years after they were recommended by Judge Pigot's advisory group on video evidence.

By the end of 2002, it was clear that full implementation of the act had been even further delayed, apparently because of a lack of resources to fund the necessary training, and, as with the Care Standards Act, it was unclear when, if ever, all of its measures would be fully implemented, and how well they would work.

But if the Longcare case highlighted one aspect of the law that needed urgent attention, it was the area of sexual offences. People with learning difficulties are so much more vulnerable to sexual assaults than those who are not learning disabled.

The law stated that it was illegal for a man to take part in a sexual act with a 'mental defective' woman (Sexual Offences Act 1956). But it was practically impossible to prove in a court that someone was a 'mental defective', and it only applied to women with severe learning difficulties. Added to that, the maximum sentence was only two years. Because prosecutors were usually unable to prove that a victim was 'mentally defective', they instead had to prove indecent assault or rape in the usual way, ie by showing the victim had not consented. There were very, very few successful prosecutions.

The problem was illustrated by the tragic case of one of 'Gordon's Girls'. After she left Longcare, she moved to a home in London. Her behaviour had been altered by the abuse she suffered at Rowe's hands. It made her more vulnerable to sexual predators and more sexually aware. She was raped by a care worker in her new home, became pregnant and had an abortion.

The judge hearing the subsequent rape case decided she had consented to the sexual acts 'by animal instinct' and the prosecution was forced to drop the case.

Members of JLS were deeply offended when they learned about the case months later. They knew the reason the woman didn't put up a struggle was that she simply didn't understand that what was being done to her was wrong, that she wasn't able to consent. There was clearly something very wrong with a legal system that allowed such an obvious miscarriage of justice.

The Home Office consultation paper *Setting the Boundaries*, which reported in July 2000, offered improvements. The paper concluded: 'We were profoundly moved by the extent of sexual abuse against vulnerable people and felt that the law needed considerable strengthening to tackle this while respecting the ability of those who could consent to sexual activity to have a private life.'

This was an important point. Introducing a law making it illegal to commit a sexual act with any person with a learning difficulty would be a dreadful restriction on their right to a sex life. So the paper recommended, firstly, that those who are not able to understand the nature or potential consequences of having sex should not be able to consent to it, and that sexual activity with such a person should be an offence, and a serious one. Secondly, there should be a new offence of a breach of a relationship of trust, banning sex between clients and their care workers. A third new criminal offence would make it illegal to obtain sex with a person with a learning difficulty by threats or deception. All three could have been applied to the crimes perpetrated by Gordon Rowe at Longcare.

These issues were highlighted again by the publication of *No Justice*, a report by Mencap, Respond and Voice UK in September 2001, which made similar recommendations. The government finally announced in November 2002 that it was intending to introduce new legislation (relying heavily on what had happened at Longcare). The bill, which began working its way through Parliament early in 2003, confirmed there would be three new sets of offences, as outlined in *Setting the Boundaries*. Firstly, it would be illegal to engage in sexual activity with a person who was unable to consent due to a learning disability, with a maximum penalty of life imprisonment. Secondly, a new offence of obtaining sexual activity with a learning disabled person by 'inducement, threat or deception' would also carry a maximum penalty of life imprisonment. And thirdly, it would be illegal for anyone working in a care setting to engage in sexual activity with a learning disabled client, with a possible 14 years in prison (a maximum sentence increased from seven years after pressure from organisations like Voice and Mencap).

Some people with milder learning difficulties were concerned about the possible criminalisation of their sex lives and outraged at the idea of courts debating whether or not they were able to consent to sex. They also feared the effect of the new laws on the people who ran and worked in care homes and day centres; they were worried that many care workers were ill-qualified to decide whether their clients were able to consent to sex, and so would tend to take the safer option of forbidding such relationships. Respond, among others, emphasised the need for staff training, even before the bill was passed.

But at least the government had listened, and sentences would for the first time reflect the seriousness of the offences. Now it was a matter of waiting for the measures to become law and hoping that, by the time they did, the criminal justice system was in a better shape to deal with such cases properly. As Voice UK's Kathryn Stone told me in May 2003, the implementation of the special measures brought in under the Youth Justice and Criminal Evidence Act had been so patchy that she feared the new laws would result in few successful prosecutions. After all, there is no point in introducing new offences, if the victims of the crimes aren't able to give their evidence.

Judge John Baker, at the end of the trial of Angela Rowe, Lorraine Field and Desmond Tully, had told the court that the Mental Health Act had provided him with inadequate sentencing powers, and that there was an urgent need for a parliamentary review of the legislation.

I called the Department of Health, which was working on a proposed new Mental Health The offences of ill-treatment and neglect are still in the draft act. And no, the maximum sentences had not been increased.

No-one, it seems, had followed through on the judge's calls. Nearly ten years on from Longcare and more than six years after the trial, this vital issue seemed to have just been forgotten. At least until the next Gordon Rowe comes along.

---

[1] Stephen O'Kell, *The Impact of Legislative Change on the Independent, Residential Care Sector*, Joseph Rowntree Foundation, 2002.
[2] Dinah Mathew, Hilary Brown, Paul Kingston, Claudine McCreadie, Janet Askham, *The Response to No Secrets; The Journal of Adult Protection*, Vol 4 Issue 1, Feb 2002.
[3] M Kebbell, S Johnson and C Hatton; *Witnesses with and without Learning Disabilities in Court: the Role of Judge Interventions*, unpublished, 2002.

Epilogue

On October 13, 2003, the day a week-long trial was due to begin at the High Court in London, Buckinghamshire County Council announced that it had finally agreed to pay compensation to the victims of the abuse at the Longcare homes. The total damages for the 54 people in the group action were expected to reach £1 million (an average of £20,000 per victim), with the council also agreeing to pay all the costs in the case. The Council refused to accept liability for what had happened at Longcare, merely agreeing that its 'shortcomings' had 'increased the risk' of abuse.

There were some brief words of regret delivered in court by Buckinghamshire's barrister, Simeon Maskrey QC, but the council's press release lacked an apology for its severe lapses and failings over a period of twenty years, and the long-term consequences they had spelled for residents at Longcare.

David Shakespeare, the leader of the council, said he was 'relieved' that an agreement had been reached. 'It is regrettable that this matter has taken so long to come to its conclusion,' he added.

I call Clare Johnson. She has an eight month old daughter, and is soon to open a nursery with her mother and sisters. She tells me she occasionally comes across former Longcare colleagues working in the industry. They now tell her the case was blown out of proportion, that it was all 'over-publicised and misrepresented'.

I go to see Dorothy and Jamie one last time. She keeps busy, taking Jamie out shopping, visiting his mother, doing the housework, and campaigning. She shows me a newspaper cutting in which she called on local businesses to do more for disabled people. She tells me she deliberately runs over produce in the aisle of the Post Office because they refuse to make it more accessible. 'I have had enough of body-abled people shoving disabled people around everywhere, just doing what they think with them.' She wants to see all residential homes closed down. 'I feel as if I have not done enough and they have not listened enough,' she says.

I ask Dorothy whether she still thinks about Longcare. 'I think about it quite a lot, but not sad thoughts,' she says. 'I think to myself if I was not a survivor in that place, if I didn't have my dreams of hope then I do not think I would have made it. Suffering like I did had its just reward in the end and its biggest reward was that that dream I held onto came true in the end. I married a man that is disabled. I have a beautiful home. There is nothing else that I want.'

More than a decade after she left Longcare, the only person she trusts is Jamie. 'He was the best thing that ever happened to me,' she says.

Although she is happy now, and she has her independent life, her husband, and her home, the memories are always there, every time she sees a non-disabled man, every time she sees a crowd of people.

Greg Adams is 'very happy' in his residential home. 'As far as anyone can tell, he is in a lifetime placement,' says Norma, his mother. 'I hope to goodness he is. He is certainly well-fed, well-housed and happy. I do not expect more than that, although I hope for more. If Greg is happy, he is successful, too, like all my other children.'

She still talks about the Longcare case. It seems almost a compulsion. 'The more people who know, the less likely it is to happen again,' she says. Her anger with the authorities for not following up her complaints properly in the early 80s has not abated. 'It took another ten years before anything was done about it,' she says. 'That evil man was allowed a further ten years to go on abusing vulnerable people.'

I visit Rosie Valton's aunt, Benedict Alcindor, a few days before Mother's Day. It was the day before Mother's Day, eight years previously, that Rosie had confided in her aunt how Rowe had raped her. 'Each Mother's Day, it just brings grief,' says Benedict. Rosie had been due to visit the previous weekend, but changed her mind and said she didn't want to come, so she will now be with Benedict and her family on the Sunday. 'I hope this

Mother's Day it will not be mentioned,' says Benedict.

Rosie still has her 'up days and down days', Benedict tells me. 'She can be cheerful when I see her, but sometimes she can be sitting there and all she will want is a hug for comfort.' Benedict believes that Rosie remembers what happened at Longcare. 'She doesn't forget her mum and she died in 1981. She remembers everything, she has a good memory.'

Nicky Power's parents, Susan and Davyd, are now on the friends committee of their daughter's home. Gordon Rowe never allowed parents to set up such an organisation at Longcare.

Her mother often turns up at Nicky's home unannounced. 'I don't phone up anymore, I just arrive.' This is good advice for other parents, she says. 'If you're in a ten or twenty-mile radius of the home, just go and do spot checks yourself.'

Nicky visits a day centre, learns social skills such as shopping, and visits the pub. She has hydrotherapy twice a week and has just started aromatherapy, but will only let the therapist touch her hands. Some of her speech is finally starting to return and she is about to begin visits to a speech therapist. For a long time, her dad was the only man she would allow near her.

Her doctor tried to take her off the tranquillisers she was prescribed to cope with her nightmares, rages and tantrums, but she just went 'back to square one', says her mum. She began to self-harm again and repeat the phrase 'not nice', which they believe refers to flashbacks to her time at Longcare. They have at least managed to wean her off the massive doses of the anti-epilepsy drug she was on at Longcare. She hasn't had a seizure since she came off the drug, so her GP believes she may never have had epilepsy.

Gary Deacon has had 'a few bad turns', but his father, Ron, hopes they are behind him now. Gary and the other residents of his current home in Slough spend most of their time sitting around with nothing to do, says Ron. 'Every time we go up there, the staff are watching television.' Neither Ron nor his wife, Doreen, believe they will find anywhere better. Ron worries about who will look after Gary once he and his wife are dead.

Gary has not had a social worker for two years. Windsor and Maidenhead Council wrote to Ron and Doreen in April 2002, saying he didn't need one because he 'now seems happy and settled in his home'. 'He should have one,' says Doreen. 'If we have queries, the home takes no notice of us.'

*

Pauline Hennessey, Janet Ward's sister, still runs a successful and very highly regarded residential home in Essex for learning disabled adults with severe challenging behaviour. She says she will only be able to keep going for another two years unless the government or Essex social services find more money to pay care home owners. Ironically, she campaigned for years for the national minimum standards brought in under the Care Standards Act, but she says the sums don't add up and good homes are going under because they can't afford to implement all the changes.

Simon Scott is happy and settled, with his DVD player, video recorder and wide-screen TV, his collection of James Bond movies, and, most importantly, his own phone. It's his 'lifeline', says Brian, his dad. 'At Stoke, you phoned them up and they would say, "oh, no, he's in bed". In the end, he didn't come to the phone at all. But at his new place, if anyone shouts at him, he phones us up and tells us to "sort 'em out".'

Simon comes home every weekend to see his mum and dad. He has IT and yoga classes at college, and attends a day centre three days a week. A physiotherapist visits him on Friday afternoons to help with his mobility.

Despite all that Simon and his parents have gone through, he also does not have his own social worker. Havering Borough Council has decided he doesn't need one because there is no record of him being ill-treated at Longcare.

The memory of Longcare seems to have faded for Simon, but not for his parents, who often attend meetings of Justice for Longcare Survivors. 'It's a hard slog,' says Brian. 'Every meeting, something comes out.' Avril agrees. 'It's very, very depressing, but now we have got to this stage, there is no way we can turn back. We just hope it will never happen again.'

Stefano Tunstell is still having behavioural problems. His psychiatrist believes they are caused by flashbacks to his time at Longcare. His parents hope music therapy will help, but they are concerned about the drugs he has been given to help his mood swings. Leslie, his father, is not sure Stefano will ever recover.

A female behavioural therapist has been working with Stefano, and seems to understand him. 'She says he must be kept very, very busy and must be taken off the drugs he was on,' says Lidia.

Although, he has a good programme of activities and a good key-worker, they want to find him a new home. 'It is very, very difficult to find the right place for him,' says Lidia. 'We are really broken-hearted. We have been looking for many places, but we have not been impressed so far.'

They worry about the future, about what will happen to their son when they are not around anymore. 'We will try to find a better home for him, but there is always change,' says Lidia. 'Suppose the director decides to sell up? What guarantee do we have that they will sell to someone who is really good and caring? When we are old and we can't do anything for him. Or when we die. There is not anyone who will look after him. His future is very, very, very bleak.'

Last year, one of the managers of the home was suspended after complaints by two care workers of possible physical abuse. Stefano came home one weekend with bruises on his wrists. The manager subsequently resigned after a multi-agency investigation including the police proved inconclusive. Lidia worries that she will simply move to a new job at another care home. She and Leslie appear bewildered and shell-shocked. It has happened again.

BIBLIOGRAPHY

Abbott, David; Morris, Jenny; and Ward, Linda: *Disabled Children and Residential Schools: A Study of Local Authority Policy and Practice*; Norah Fry Research Centre, supported by Joseph Rowntree Foundation, 2000

Atkinson, Dorothy; Jackson, Mark; and Walmsley, Jan: *Forgotten Lives: Exploring the History of Learning Disability*; bild; 1997

Boston, Sarah: *Too Deep for Tears—Eighteen Years after the Death of Will, My Son*; London: Pandora, 1994

Boyle, Mike and Leadbetter, Mike: *Enough is Enough*; Elite Recruitment Specialists, 1998

Brown, Hilary; Stein, June; and Turk, Vicky: *The Sexual Abuse of Adults with Learning Disabilities: Report Of A Second Two-Year Incidence Survey*; Mental Handicap Research, Vol 8, No 1, 1995

Brown, Hilary; Stein, June: *Implementing Adult Protection Policies in Kent and East Sussex*; Journal of Social Policy, 27, 3, 1998

Brown, Hilary; Stein, June: *Monitoring Adult Protection Referrals in 10 English Local Authorities*; The Journal of Adult Protection, Vol 2, Issue 3, September 2000

Burgner, Tom; Russell, Dr Philippa; Whitehead, Simon; Tinnion, John: *Independent Longcare Inquiry*; Buckinghamshire County Council, June 1998

Burke, Lillian; Bedard, Cheryl: *Self-injury Considered in Association with Sexual Victimization in Individuals with a Developmental Handicap*; The Canadian Journal of Human Sexuality, Vol 3(3), Autumn 1994

Cole, Sandra: *Preface to the Special Issue on Sexual Exploitation of Persons with Disabilities*; Sexuality and Disability, Vol 9, No 3, 1991

Collins, Jean: *The Resettlement Game: policy and procrastination in the closure of mental handicap hospitals*; Values Into Action, supported by Joseph Rowntree Foundation, 1993

Craft, Ann; Hitching, Marjorie: *Keeping Safe: Sex Education and Assertiveness Skills*;

Thinking the Unthinkable, papers on Sexual Abuse and People with Learning Difficulties: eds Brown, Hilary and Craft, Ann; Family Planning Association Education Unit, 1989

DHSS and Welsh Office: *Better Services for the Mentally Handicapped*, Government White Paper, 1971

Diesfield, Kate: *Witness Credibility in Cases of Sexual Abuse Against Adults with Learning Disabilities*; Tizard Learning Disability Review, Volume 1 Issue 4

Diplock, Monica: *The History of Leavesden Hospital*, 1990

Dunne, Timothy; Power, Anne: *Sexual Abuse and Mental Handicap: Preliminary Findings of a Community-based Study*; Mental Handicap Research, 1990, 3:2

Eden, D J: *Mental Handicap: An Introduction*; Allen and U, 1976

Gunn, Michael: *Sexual Abuse and Adults with Mental Handicap: Can the Law Help?*; Thinking the Unthinkable, papers on Sexual Abuse and People with Learning Difficulties: eds Brown, Hilary and Craft, Ann; Family Planning Association Education Unit, 1989

Home Office: consultation paper: *Setting the Boundaries—Reforming the Law on Sexual Offences*, July 2000

Jackson, Robin (ed): *Bound to Care, An Anthology—Family Experiences of Mental Handicap*; Rescare, 1996

Judicial Studies Board: *Equal Treatment Bench Book*, October 2000

Kilgallon W; Day, Dr K; Robinson, N; Community Healthcare North Durham: *Report of external review panel into the process and robustness of Community Health Care: North Durham NHS Trust's handling of untoward incidents and the investigation into the learning disabilities service at Earls House Hospital*, February 1998

Law Commission Report No 231: *Mental Incapacity*, 1995

Malster, Robert: *St Lawrence's: The Story of a Hospital, 1870-1994*; Lifecare NHS Trust, 1994

Mathew, Dinah; Brown, Hilary; Kingston, Paul; McCreadie, Claudine; Askham, Janet: *The Response to No Secrets*; The Journal of Adult Protection, Vol 4, Issue 1, February 2002

McCarthy, Michelle; Thompson, David: *A Prevalence Study of Sexual Abuse of Adults with Intellectual Disabilities Referred for Sex Education*; Journal of Applied Research in Intellectual Disabilities, Vol 10, No 2, 1997

McCarthy, Michelle: *Sexual Violence against Women with Learning Disabilities*; Feminism and Psychology, Vol 8(4), 1998

McCarthy, Michelle: Consent, *Abuse and Choices—Women with Intellectual Disabilities and Sexuality*; from Traustadottir, R and Johnson, K (eds): *Women with Intellectual Disabilities: Finding a Place in the World*; 2000; Jessica Kingsley

McGowan, Chandra: *A Long Way from Home*; The Health Service Journal; April 25, 1996

Mencap: *Barriers to Justice—A Mencap study into how the criminal justice system treats people with learning disabilities*, November 1997

Morris, Pauline: *Put Away, A Sociological Study of Institutions for the Mentally Retarded;* Routledge and Kegan Paul, 1969

North West Training and Development Team: *Sexual Abuse and People with Learning Disabilities—report of a conference held on 18 October 1995 at Bolton*

Potts, Maggie; and Fido, Rebecca: *A Fit Person to be Removed: Personal Accounts of Life in a Mental Deficiency Institution;* Northcote House, 1991

Pritchard, D G: *Education and the Handicapped: 1760-1960;* Routledge and Kegan Paul, 1963

Report of the Committee of Inquiry into Allegations of Ill-Treatment of Patients and other irregularities at the Ely Hospital, Cardiff; HMSO, March 1969

Report of the Committee of Inquiry into Normansfield Hospital; HMSO, November 1978

Report of the Committee of Inquiry into South Ockendon Hospital; HMSO; May 1974

Report of the Farleigh Hospital Committee of Inquiry; HMSO, April 1971

Reynolds, Leigh Ann: *People with Mental Retardation and Sexual Abuse;* (Internet)

Richardson, M: *Reflection and Celebration—Neal (1960-1987): Narrative of a Young Man with Profound and Multiple Disabilities;* Journal of Learning Disabilities for Nursing, Health and Social Care, (1997) 1(4)

Rushton, Alan; Beaumont, Kay; and Mayes, Debbie: *Service and Client Outcomes of Cases Reported Under a Joint Vulnerable Adults Policy;* The Journal of Adult Protection, Vol 2, Issue 2, June 2000

Sanders, Andrew; Creaton, Jane; Bird, Sophia; and Weber, Leanne: *Home Office Research and Statistics Directorate, Research Findings No 44—Witnesses with Learning Disabilities*

Sellin, Birger: *In Dark Hours I Find My Way—messages from an autistic mind;* London: Victor Gollancz, 1993

Sinason, Valerie: *Secondary Mental Handicap and its Relationship to Trauma;* Psychoanalytic Psychotherapy (1986), Vol 2 No 2

Sinason, Valerie: *Uncovering and Responding to Sexual Abuse in Psychotherapeutic Settings; Thinking the Unthinkable, papers on Sexual Abuse and People with Learning Difficulties:* eds Brown, Hilary and Craft, Ann; Family Planning Association Education Unit, 1989

Sobsey, Dick; and Doe, Tanis: *Patterns of Sexual Abuse and Assault;* Sexuality and Disability, Vol 9, No 3, 1991

Social Services Inspectorate, Department of Health: *Inspection of Local Authority Social Services Department Inspection Units: Buckinghamshire,* May 1995

Social Services Inspectorate for Wales: *Social Services in Wales 1999-2000—The Report of the Chief Inspector,* January 2001

Speaking Up For Justice—Report of the Interdepartmental Working Group on the Treatment of Vulnerable or Intimidated Witnesses in the Criminal Justice System, June 1998

Stanley, Nicky; Manthorpe, Jill; and Penhale, Bridget (Eds): *Institutional Abuse— perspectives across the life course;* Routledge, 1999

Tsuchiya, Takashi: *Eugenic Sterilizations in Japan and Recent Demands for an Apology: A Report*; Ethics and Intellectual Disability, Vol 3, No 1, Autumn 1997

Varley, Christopher: *Schizophreniform Psychoses in Mentally Retarded Adolescent Girls Following Sexual Assault*; American Journal of Psychiatry, April 1984

Walmsley, Sandra: *The Need for Safeguards*; Thinking the Unthinkable, papers on Sexual Abuse and People with Learning Difficulties, eds Brown, Hilary and Craft, Ann; Family Planning Association Education Unit, 1989

Wetherall, Grant: *Investigation of Abuse of People with Learning Disabilities at Stoke Poges, Buckinghamshire*; practice study for diploma in social work, Brunel University, June 1995

Williams, Christopher: *Invisible Victims—crime and abuse against people with learning disabilities*; London: Jessica Kingsley Publishers, 1995

Wright, David and Digby, Anne (eds): *From Idiocy to Mental Deficiency—Historical Perspectives on People with Learning Disabilities*; Routledge, 1996:

Digby, Anne: *Contexts and Pespectives*

Neugebauer, Richard: *Mental Handicap in Medieval and Early Modern England: Criteria, Measurement and Care*

Rushton, Peter: *Idiocy, the Family and the Community in Early Modern North-East England*

Andrews, Jonathan: *Identifying and Providing for the Mentally Disabled in Early Modern London*

(Goodey, C F: *The Psychopolitics of Learning and Disability in Seventeenth-Century Thought*)

Wright, David: *'Childlike in his Innocence': Lay Attitudes to 'Idiots' and 'Imbeciles' in Victorian England*

Gladstone, David: *The Changing Dynamic of Institutional Care: The Western Counties Idiot Asylum, 1864-1914*

Jackson, Mark: *Institutional Provision for the Feeble-Minded in Edwardian England: Sandlebridge and the Scientific Morality of Permanent Care*

Cox, Pamela: *Girls, Deficiency and Delinquency*

Thomson, Mathew: *Family, Community, and State: The Micro-Politics of Mental Deficiency*

ORGANISATIONS

Central England People First:
www.peoplefirst.org.uk

National Autistic Society:
Helpline 0870 600 8585 (Mon to Fri, 10am to 4pm)
www.nas.org.uk

Mencap:
Helpline 0808 808 1111
www.mencap.org.uk

Public Concern At Work:
UK helpline 020 7404 6609 or email helpline@pcaw.co.uk
Scotland helpline 0141 5507572 or email scot@pcaw.co.uk
www.pcaw.co.uk

Respond:
Helpline 0808 808 0700 (Mon to Fri, 1.30pm to 5pm)
www.respond.org.uk

Voice UK:
Tel 01332 202555
www.voiceuk.clara.net

Ms Ali O'Callaghan and Professor Glynis Murphy
The Tizard Centre
Beverley Farm
University of Kent
Canterbury CT2 7LZ
email A.C.OCallaghan@ukc.ac.uk
and g.h.murphy@ukc.ac.uk

Dr Isabel Clare
Department of Psychiatry (Section of Developmental Psychiatry)
Douglas House
18b Trumpington Road
Cambridge CB2 2AH
email ichc2@hermes.cam.ac.uk

Disability Now (newspaper)
Disability Now
6 Market Road
London N7 9PW
editor@disabilitynow.org.uk
www.disabilitynow.org.uk

INDEX

Abbott, Dorothy: 13-5, 43-5, 69-70, 89-90, 117, 125, 149, 157-8, 184-8, 197, 229-30
Abuse,
    General: 25, 35, 42, 45, 49, 55-6, 73, 171-4, 180-4, 96
    Neglect: 23, 24, 25, 59, 79, 83, 99, 117, 124, 127, 133, 136, 144, 147, 149, 153, 159, 167, 183, 184, 227
    Physical: 14, 56, 67, 69, 70, 74, 76, 81, 87, 90-2, 96, 99, 103-4, 112, 117, 118, 119, 127, 137, 147, 154, 155-6, 162, 166, 171-2, 174, 177, 179, 187, 198, 199, 204, 208, 210, 212
    Sexual: 15, 30, 51-2, 53, 54, 61, 69, 65, 69, 72, 74, 75, 87, 89, 92, 93-4, 95, 96, 97, 98, 99, 100, 104, 124, 127-8, 114, 117, 118, 119, 133, 137, 143, 144-5, 147, 152, 153, 162, 163, 166, 171-2, 173, 174, 179, 180, 182-4, 187, 188, 193, 195, 204, 211, 221, 224-6, 231
'Animal instincts' and rape: 225

Boateng, Paul: 16, 122
Broadmoor: 50-1, 55, 56-7, 61, 67, 80, 82, 83, 91, 92, 107, 134, 142

Drugs: 23, 31, 54, 56, 59, 82-3, 95, 137, 142-6, 148, 151, 154, 181-2, 191, 203-4, 207, 211, 232, 233
    contraception: 140, 141, 142, 145, 203
    Haloperidol: 144
    Largactil: 59, 83, 182
    medication: 14, 119, 138, 140, 142, 145, 146, 149, 152, 161, 184, 185, 195, 200, 214
    sedatives: 31, 56, 142, 143, 146, 149
    tranquilisers: 24, 60, 144, 182, 191, 210, 231

Eugenics: 21, 33-4, 170

Fraud: 72, 84-6, 87-9, 118, 119, 128
long-stay hospitals: 22-24, 25, 29, 34, 37, 38, 45, 61, 65, 156, 158, 159, 167, 181, 185, 216, 222

Mactaggart, Fiona: 16, 164, 222-3

Mencap: 25, 41, 42, 60, 116, 180-1, 213, 218-9, 226,

Mental Deficiency Act (1913): 21, 34

Mental Health Act (1959): 22, 127, 155, 226-7

People First: 25, 52, 175-80, 216

Police: 25, 45, 49, 52-4, 58, 60-2, 66, 68, 78-9, 87, 89, 92, 95, 100, 106, 110, 111, 113-5, 117, 118-9, 121-2, 124-30, 131-3, 135, 140, 145, 146, 150-3, 155, 164, 169-70, 177, 178, 181, 183, 188, 192, 193, 210, 214-5, 220-1, 223-4, 234

Rowe, Gordon
    Abuse, sexual: 15, 52, 53, 54, 61, 65, 87, 93-5, 96, 97, 98, 99, 100, 104, 114, 117, 119, 124, 127, 131, 133, 142, 143, 153, 174, 162, 163, 171, 195, 231
    Abuse, verbal: 73-4, 96
Russell, Dr Philippa: 17, 145-6, 151, 164, 172, 174-5

Scope: 36, 186
secure unit: 143
Setting the Boundaries, Reforming the Law on Sex Offences (2000): 58, 92, 225, 226
Sexual Offences Act (1956): 225

Thatcher, Margaret: 57

Valuing People, A New Strategy for Learning Disability for the 21st Century (2001): 29, 37, 74, 170, 178, 179, 218, 219, 222
Voice UK: 213, 223, 226